Persistent Depressive Disorders

T0315317

About the Author

J. Kim Penberthy, PhD, ABPP, is the Chester F. Carlson Professor of Psychiatry & Neurobehavioral Sciences at the University of Virginia School of Medicine in Charlottesville, VA. She has spent her career treating patients with depressive disorders, training other professionals regarding effective treatments, and conducting research in the effective diagnosis and treatment of depression and related disorders. Dr. Penberthy is internationally known for her research regarding effective treatment for persistent depression and related disorders using the cognitive behavioral analysis system of psychotherapy (CBASP) and has developed applications for comorbidities and group administration.

Advances in Psychotherapy – Evidence-Based Practice

Series Editor
Danny Wedding, PhD, MPH, Saybrook University, Oakland, CA

Associate Editors
Larry Beutler, PhD, Professor, Palo Alto University / Pacific Graduate School of Psychology, Palo Alto, CA
Kenneth E. Freedland, PhD, Professor of Psychiatry and Psychology, Washington University School of Medicine, St. Louis, MO
Linda C. Sobell, PhD, ABPP, Professor, Center for Psychological Studies, Nova Southeastern University, Ft. Lauderdale, FL
David A. Wolfe, PhD, ABPP, Adjunct Professor, Faculty of Education, Western University, London, ON

The basic objective of this series is to provide therapists with practical, evidence-based treatment guidance for the most common disorders seen in clinical practice – and to do so in a reader-friendly manner. Each book in the series is both a compact "how-to" reference on a particular disorder for use by professional clinicians in their daily work and an ideal educational resource for students as well as for practice-oriented continuing education.

The most important feature of the books is that they are practical and easy to use: All are structured similarly and all provide a compact and easy-to-follow guide to all aspects that are relevant in real-life practice. Tables, boxed clinical "pearls," marginal notes, and summary boxes assist orientation, while checklists provide tools for use in daily practice.

Continuing Education Credits

Psychologists and other healthcare providers may earn five continuing education credits for reading the books in the *Advances in Psychotherapy* series and taking a multiple-choice exam. This continuing education program is a partnership of Hogrefe Publishing and the National Register of Health Service Psychologists. Details are available at https://us.hogrefe.com/cenatreg

The National Register of Health Service Psychologists is approved by the American Psychological Association to sponsor continuing education for psychologists. The National Register maintains responsibility for this program and its content.

Advances in Psychotherapy – Evidence-Based Practice, Volume 43

Persistent Depressive Disorders

J. Kim Penberthy
University of Virginia, Charlottesville, VA

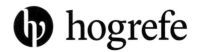

Library of Congress Cataloging in Publication information for the print version of this book
is available via the Library of Congress Marc Database under the Library of Congress Control
Number 2019933086

Library and Archives Canada Cataloguing in Publication

Title: Persistent depressive disorders / J. Kim Penberthy, University of Virginia, Charlottesville, VA.
Names: Penberthy, J. Kim, author.
Series: Advances in psychotherapy--evidence-based practice ; v. 43.
Description: Series statement: Advances in psychotherapy--evidence-based practice ; volume 43 |
    Includes bibliographical references.
Identifiers: Canadiana (print) 20190060794 | Canadiana (ebook) 20190060808 | ISBN 9780889375055
    (softcover) | ISBN 9781616765057 (PDF) | ISBN 9781613345054 (EPUB)
Subjects: LCSH: Depression, Mental—Treatment—Handbooks, manuals, etc. | LCSH: Depression, Mental—
    Diagnosis—Handbooks, manuals, etc. | LCSH: Depression, Mental—Etiology—Handbooks, manuals, etc.
    | LCGFT: Handbooks and manuals.
Classification: LCC RC537 P46 2019 | DDC 616.85/27—dc23

© 2019 by Hogrefe Publishing
http://www.hogrefe.com

PUBLISHING OFFICES

USA: Hogrefe Publishing Corporation, 7 Bulfinch Place, Suite 202, Boston, MA 02114
                Phone (866) 823-4726, Fax (617) 354-6875; E-mail customerservice@hogrefe.com
EUROPE: Hogrefe Publishing GmbH, Merkelstr. 3, 37085 Göttingen, Germany
                Phone +49 551 99950-0, Fax +49 551 99950-111; E-mail publishing@hogrefe.com

SALES & DISTRIBUTION

USA: Hogrefe Publishing, Customer Services Department,
                30 Amberwood Parkway, Ashland, OH 44805
                Phone (800) 228-3749, Fax (419) 281-6883; E-mail customerservice@hogrefe.com
UK: Hogrefe Publishing, c/o Marston Book Services Ltd., 160 Eastern Ave.,
                Milton Park, Abingdon, OX14 4SB, UK
                Phone +44 1235 465577, Fax +44 1235 465556; E-mail direct.orders@marston.co.uk
EUROPE: Hogrefe Publishing, Merkelstr. 3, 37085 Göttingen, Germany
                Phone +49 551 99950-0, Fax +49 551 99950-111; E-mail publishing@hogrefe.com

OTHER OFFICES

CANADA: Hogrefe Publishing, 660 Eglinton Ave. East, Suite 119-514, Toronto, Ontario, M4G 2K2
SWITZERLAND: Hogrefe Publishing, Länggass-Strasse 76, 3012 Bern

ISBN 978-0-88937-505-5 (print) • ISBN 978-1-61676-505-7 (PDF) • ISBN 978-1-61334-505-4 (EPUB)
http://doi.org/10.1027/00505-000

Contents

1

Description of Persistent Depressive Disorders

1.1   Terminology

The American Psychiatric Association (APA) *Diagnostic and Statistical Manual of Mental Disorders*, fifth edition (DSM-5; APA, 2013) lists eight distinct depressive disorders, with the common feature of all being the presence of sad, empty, or irritable mood, accompanied by somatic and cognitive changes that negatively impact functioning. What differs among these depressive disorders is chronicity, timing of symptoms, and presumed etiology. This book will focus on the DSM-5 category of **persistent depressive disorder** (PDD), which is an amalgamation of the categories from the DSM, fourth edition (DSM-IV; APA, 1994), of **dysthymic disorder** (DD), chronic **major depressive disorder** (MDD), and DD with a **major depressive episode** (MDE) also referred to as **double depression**

Persistent depressive disorder is a newly named category in DSM-5 that integrates DD and MDD

PDD and DD are both coded as 300.4 in the DSM-5. In the International Classification of Diseases, 10th edition, PDD is coded as F34.1 and Dysthymic Disorder is coded as 6A72 in the ICD-11 (ICD-10, WHO, 1992; ICD-11, WHO, 2018). The DSM-5 code for MDE is 296.XX with extensions to distinguish recurrence and severity (unspecified 296.X0, mild 296.X1, moderate 296.X2, severe with psychotic features 296.X4 or without psychotic features 296.X3, full 296.X6 or partial remission 296.X5) and identifiers that specify with anxious distress, mixed features, melancholic features, atypical features, mood-congruent psychotic features, mood-incongruent psychotic features, peripartum onset, catatonia (for which there are the additional DSM-5 code 293.89 and ICD-10 code F06.1), and seasonal pattern (used with recurrent episodes only). The ICD-10 code for MDE, single episode, is F32.X and recurrent MDE is coded as F33.X, with severity extensions (mild F3X.0, moderate F3X.1, severe F3X.2, with psychotic features F3X.3, unspecified F3X.9, and partial F3X.4 or full remission F3X.5). Other specifiers include early onset (onset prior to age 21 years) or late onset (onset at age 21 years or older). The ICD-11 code for single episode depressive disorder is 6A70 and recurrent depressive disorder is coded as 6A71 (WHO, 2018). The ICD-11 also has a diagnostic code for mixed depressive and anxiety disorder where neither sets of symptoms, considered separately would justify a depression or anxiety diagnosis, but symptoms are present and impair functioning (WHO, 2018).

1.2   Definition

Researchers have found few meaningful differences between DD and chronic MDD (Keller et al., 1995; Klein & Santiago, 2003), and thus these were merged into PDD in DSM-5. This new category of depressive disorders gives more weight to duration than to severity of symptoms. DSM-5 defines PDD using the same set of symptoms as that used for DD, with the assumption that most patients who meet the full criteria for chronic MDD also meet the criteria for DD. However, because of differences in symptomatic criteria, especially regarding duration of symptoms, some patients with chronic MDD will not meet the DSM-5 criteria for PDD. The diagnosis of PDD in DSM-5 includes both chronic MDD and DD as defined by the DSM-IV (APA, 1994), and provides specifiers that define the combination between these two conditions. Thus, the diagnosis of PDD is indicated if any of the following are present:

- PDD as pure DD with no MDE during a 2-year period;
- Double depression: PDD with intermittent MDEs, where the criteria for one or more MDEs have been met during a 2-year period of DD, but the symptoms did not reach the diagnostic threshold of MDE for at least 8 weeks;
- PDD and chronic MDD (MDE criteria have been met for > 2 years) both diagnosed;
- Chronic MDD only where the MDD has been present for > 2 years.

Figure 1 provides a visual representation of these course profiles.

PDD is characterized by depressed mood that occurs for most of the day, for more days than not, for a duration of at least 2 years in an adult, or at least 1 year in a child or adolescent. Children or adolescents may experience irritability instead of depressed mood. During periods of depressed mood or irritability, at least two of six additional symptoms listed in Box 1 must be present to diagnosis PDD, and any symptom-free intervals must last no longer than 2 months to maintain the diagnosis of PDD. Additionally, there must never have been a manic, mixed, or hypomanic episode in the first 2 years, and criteria must never have been met for cyclothymic disorder. To meet the diagnostic criteria for PDD, the symptoms must not be due to the direct physiological effects of the use or abuse of a substance (e.g., alcohol, illicit drugs, or medications), a general medical condition (such as cancer or a stroke), or be better explained by the patient meeting criteria for schizoaffective disorder, schizophrenia, delusional disorder, or other psychotic disorder. The symptoms must also cause significant distress or impairment in social, occupational, educational, and/or other important areas of functioning.

Children or adolescents may endorse irritability instead of depressed mood

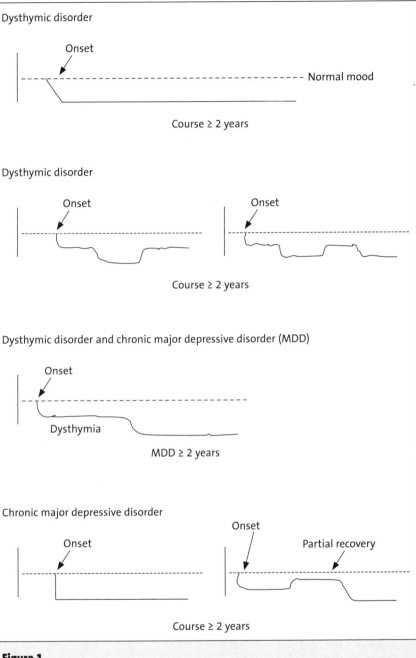

Figure 1
Course profiles of persistent depressive disorders. Reprinted with permission from unpublished material by James P. McCullough, Jr., 2018.
MDD = major depressive disorder.

Box 1
Summary of DSM-5 Diagnostic Criteria for Persistent Depressive Disorder or Dysthymic Disorder

- Depressed mood most of day, more days than not for 2 years. Adolescents or children may have irritable mood for 1 year.
- While depressed, must have two or more of the following:
  - Poor or increased appetite or eating
  - Insomnia or hypersomnia
  - Low energy or fatigue
  - Low self-esteem
  - Concentration or decision-making difficulties
  - Hopelessness
- Must not be without symptoms for more than 2 months
- MDD may be present for 2 years
- No mania or hypomania present
- Symptoms cause functional impairment or distress
- Symptoms not better explained by other psychiatric disorder, effects of substances, or medical condition

Note. For full diagnostic criteria, see APA (2013), pp. 168–169. MDD = major depressive disorder.

PDD patients who also meet MDD criteria for 2 years should be given a diagnosis of both PDD and MDD

The 2-year minimum duration has been debated, and researchers examining characteristics of DD in adults occasionally use symptom duration of 1 year or longer (Brown, Craig, & Harris, 2008). For clinical and prognostic purposes, the duration of depressive symptoms is important both below and above the 2-year mark regardless of criteria met. MDD may precede PDD, and MDEs may occur during PDD. Patients who meet MDD criteria for 2 years should be given a diagnosis of PDD as well as MDD.

The diagnostic criteria for an MDE are listed in Box 2. To have a diagnosis of MDE, the patient must endorse having five or more of the nine symptoms within the same 2-week period, with at least one of the symptoms being depressed mood or loss of interest or pleasure. The other caveats for diagnosis of MDE are the same as those for PDD. The diagnosis of MDD is made if criteria for MDE are continually met for at least 2 years, and there is a lifetime absence of mania and hypomania.

Box 2
Summary of DSM-5 Diagnostic Criteria for a Major Depressive Episode

- Five or more symptoms are present for 2 weeks, and they are a change from previous functioning. At least one of the symptoms must be depressed mood or lack or loss of interest or pleasure
- Criteria for MDE may be present continuously for 2 years or more, and that would be a separate diagnosis from PDD
- Possible symptoms include all of those in PDD as well as:
  - Decreased interest or pleasure in activities or things
  - Physical or psychomotor agitation or slowness
  - Feelings of worthless or guilt which are not warranted
  - Recurrent thoughts of death, or suicidal ideation, plan, or attempt

Note. For full diagnostic criteria, see APA (2013), pp. 160–161. MDE = major depressive episode; PDD = persistent depressive disorder.

If all of the symptoms of MDE are present during a PDD, an additional diagnosis of MDE should be made – this is sometimes referred to as double depression. An additional important change in DSM-5 is that bereavement is not excluded from the MDE diagnostic criteria, as it was in DSM-IV, meaning that it is possible for patients with mild to moderate symptoms of depression to be diagnosed with MDE within the first 2 months following a loved one's death.

Some researchers have proposed that the relabeling of chronic MDD and DD into the diagnosis of PDD risks the creation of another broad and heterogeneous diagnosis and have hypothesized that DD is best defined as a type of depression experienced within MDD (Rhebergen & Graham, 2014). Others have provided evidence supporting the idea that persistent or chronic depression is a specific diagnostic subtype within the larger group of affective disorders (Rubio, Markowitz, & Alegria, 2011). McCullough et al. (1990) emphasized the distinction between early-onset (depression before the age of 21 years) and late-onset (depression at or after the age of 21) patients as proposed by Akiskal et al. (Akiskal, King, Rosenthal, Robinson, & Scott-Strauss, 1981). This distinction is substantiated by evidence that the majority of patients with DD (72%) have an early onset and that these patients have an earlier onset of MDE with a longer index of the initial MDE, which suggests a more severe condition (Klein et al., 1999).

> An MDD diagnosis is made if MDE symptoms are continually met for at least 2 years
>
> If symptoms of an MDE are present during PDD, both disorders are diagnosed; called double depression
>
> In DSM-5, bereavement is not excluded from MDE diagnosis, as it was in DSM-IV
>
> Seventy-two percent of patients with DD have an early onset

1.3   Epidemiology

Data regarding prevalence of PDD can be confusing due to changes in the DSM-5 criteria and the fact that some epidemiological surveys document and record MDEs, and others use chronic MDD, and still others use DD or PDD as their criteria. Double depression is not always specified in studies evaluating rates of depression. Thus, current rates of depression may vary from past reports, and care should be used in interpreting data.

The WHO (WHO, 2017) categorizes depression as DD, MDE, or MDD in their epidemiological research, and as such may be an overestimate of PDD as described in the DSM-5. The WHO (2017) estimates that as of 2015, there were 322 million people worldwide diagnosed with DD, MDE, or MDD, which is an 18% increase since 2005. The WHO ranks depression as the leading cause of ill health and disability worldwide, and estimates global rates of depression at 4.4%, with depression being more common among females (5.1%) than males (3.6%). Prevalence varies by WHO region, from a low of 2.6% among adult males in the Western Pacific Region and 5.9% among adult females in the African Region. Prevalence rates also vary by age, peaking in older adulthood (about 7.5% among women aged 55–74 years, and about 5.5% among men in the same age group).

> WHO ranked depression as the leading cause of ill health and disability worldwide

About 20% of adult patients who have an MDE suffer from chronic MDD (Angst, Gamma, Rossler, Ajdacic, & Klein, 2009), which is defined as meeting criteria for MDE continually for at least 2 years. The 12-month prevalence and lifetime prevalence for chronic MDD has been estimated to be 5.3% and 13.2%, respectively (Hasin, Goodwin, Stinson, & Grant, 2005). A review of

DSM-5 cites a 12-month prevalence rate of 7% for MDD

DSM-5 cites a 12-month prevalence rate of 0.5% for PDD

prior studies up to the year 2000 found a 12-month prevalence rate of 4.1% and an average lifetime prevalence rate of 6.7% for MDD (Waraich, Goldner, Somers, & Hsu, 2004). The DSM-5 cites data from the Kessler et al. (2003) study, which gives a 12-month prevalence rate of 7% for MDD in the US.

Multiple studies have explored the prevalence of DD in the US using the DSM-IV criteria. The National Comorbidity Survey–Replication reported a 12-month DD prevalence of 1.5% (Kessler et al., 2003). The DSM-5 cites 12-month prevalence rates of 0.5% for PDD based on data from Blanco et al. (2010). In a 2004 analysis of the literature, investigators determined a lifetime prevalence of 3.6% for DD in US communities (Waraich et al., 2004).

In a recent study of the prevalence of DSM-5–specified MDD and related disorders, researchers determined a lifetime prevalence of 15.2% for PDD with persistent MDD, 3.3% for PDD with pure DD, and 28.3% for any report of MDE or MDD (Vandeleur et al., 2017). These same researchers reported that patients with PDD and MDD were the most severely impaired, followed by those with recurrent MDE, single episode MDE, and PDD. They further suggest that this research casts doubt on the pertinence of grouping MDD and DD within the new category of PDD. These data may explain higher reported prevalence rates of MDD when both MDE and MDD are combined in one group. A summary of lifetime prevalence rates from Vandeleur et al. (2017) is shown in Table 1.

Fewer studies of the incidence of PDD and MDD are available. Waraich, Goldner, Somers, and Hsu (2004) conducted a review including incidence rates of mood disorders and found only four studies exploring annual incidence rates of MDD. Those authors provided an overall best estimate incidence rate of 2.9 per 100 with a 95% confidence interval (95% CI) of 1.3 to 4.8. These

Table 1
Lifetime Prevalence of Persistent Depressive Disorder

	Lifetime prevalence (95% CI)	Male (95% CI)	Female (95% CI)
Any MDD or MDE	28.0 (26.5–29.4)	21.5 (19.6–23.4)	33.7 (31.6–35.8)
MDE, single episode	17.4 (16.2–18.6)	14.6 (12.9–16.2)	20.0 (18.2–21.7)
MDE, recurrent episodes	10.6 (10.0–11.5)	6.9 (5.7–8.1)	13.8 (12.2–15.3)
PDD with chronic MDD	15.2 (14.1–16.4)	10.2 (8.8–11.7)	19.6 (17.9–21.4)
PDD as pure DD	2.5 (2.0–3.0)	1.9 (1.3–2.5)	3.0 (2.2–3.8)
PDD with intermittent MDE (double depression)	0.4 (0.2–0.5)	0.3 (0.1–0.6)	0.4 (0.0–0.6)

Note. CI = confidence interval; DD = dysthymic disorder; MDD = major depressive disorder; MDE = major depressive episode; PDD = persistent depressive disorder. Adapted from "Prevalence and Correlates of DSM-5 Major Depressive and Related Disorders in the Community," by C. L. Vandeleur et al., 2017, *Psychiatry Research, 250*, pp. 50–58. © 2017 by Psychiatry Research.

results are fairly old and quite variable and thus should be interpreted with caution. Angst et al. (2009) prospectively studied a group of people in Zurich and found a 5.7% cumulative incidence rate for what they termed "long-term depression" which was a combination of DD, MDD, and double depression diagnoses.

1.3.1 Gender and Sex Differences

Epidemiological studies have shown that the lifetime prevalence of both DD and MDD in women is almost twice that in men (Blanco et al., 2010). This ratio has been documented in different countries and across ethnic groups. A comprehensive review of almost all general population studies conducted to date in the US, Puerto Rico, Canada, France, Iceland, Taiwan, Korea, Germany, and Hong Kong, reported that women predominate over men in life-time prevalence rates of major depression (Piccinelli & Gomez Homen, 1997). This difference has been documented in clinical and community samples and across racial groups. Depression may be more persistent in women, and female sex is a significant predictor of relapse (Kuehner, 1999). Sex differences relating to depression vary with age, with male and female children showing similar incidence rates. Sex differences in prevalence rates first appear around the age of 10 years and persist until midlife, after which they disappear (Noble, 2005). Therefore, women have the greatest risk for developing depressive disorders during their childbearing years. Before puberty and after menopause in women, the two sexes appear to be affected about equally (Noble, 2005).

> DD and MDD are approximately twice as common among females than males worldwide

Several biological processes are thought to be involved in the predisposition of women to depression, including genetically determined vulnerability, hormonal fluctuations related to various aspects of reproductive function, and sensitivity to such hormonal fluctuations in brain systems that mediate depressive states. Psychosocial events such as role-stress, victimization, sex-specific socialization, internalization coping style, and disadvantaged social status may all contribute to the increased vulnerability of women to depression. Depression in women may develop during different phases of the reproductive cycle, and infertility, miscarriage, oral contraceptives, and hormone replacement treatment have been associated with depression in women (Noble, 2005).

In a systematic review and meta-analysis, Lucassen, Stasiak, Samra, Frampton, and Merry (2017) reported robust evidence that rates of depressive disorders are elevated in sexual minority youths in comparison with heterosexual young people. Their research demonstrated that sexual minority youths have approximately 2 times the odds of a depressive disorder compared with their heterosexual peers. They further state that female sexual minority youths appear to be at particular risk. In a review of PDD in transgender versus cisgender patients, in both adults and adolescents, Budge, Adelson, and Howard (2013) found MDE rates of 51.4% for transgender women and 48.3% for transgender men – rates that far surpass those for the general population. Additional research supports this finding, with lifetime prevalence rates of MDD or DD for transgender patients, ranging from 48% to 62% (Nemoto, Bodeker, & Iwamoto, 2011; Nuttbrock et al., 2010). Even after sexual reassignment procedures to alleviate gender dysphoria, depressive disorders often

> Rates of MDD and DD are significantly higher in sexual minority populations

persist in this population (Dhejne et al., 2011). Sadly, there are also high rates of attempted suicide, with 32% of both transgender men and women ever having attempted suicide (Clements-Nolle, Marx, Guzman, & Katz, 2001).

Theories regarding why rates of PDD are so high among sexual minorities include minority stress theory, which posits that patients who have minority identities may experience stress and related depressive symptoms due to experiences of discrimination and aggression (Budge et al., 2013; Nuttbrock et al., 2014). Nuttbrock et al. (2014) found a significant association between gender abuse and MDE in transgender females. Budge et al. (2013) found that avoidant coping served as a mediator between transition status and depressive symptoms in a group of transgender patients, where transition status was negatively related to avoidant coping. The further along patients were in their identity process, the less avoidant coping they used. Those who used more avoidant coping strategies reported more depression and anxiety. Budge et al. (2013) hypothesized that those patients who are in the beginning stages of their transition process may use more avoidant coping, and thus are at increased risk for depressive disorders.

1.3.2   Age

Point prevalence rates of MDD or DD in childhood are approximately 1–3%

MDD may first appear at any age, but the likelihood of onset generally increases with puberty, with the incidence peaking in the 20s. Point prevalence estimates of MDD are low in childhood at about 1% to 3%, but by adolescence, the rates are comparable to those found in adulthood (Kessler et al., 2005). Patients with adolescent-onset MDD experience more negative outcomes relative to nondepressed adolescents or those with adult-onset MDD (Lewinsohn, Hops, Roberts, Seeley, & Andrews, 1993). The Oregon Adolescent Depression Project (Lewinsohn, et al., 1993) was a prospective, epidemiological study of adolescents assessed through age 30. These researchers found that the natural course of adolescent-onset MDD is marked by impairment in a range of important psychosocial domains, including relationship quality, school and work functioning, finances, physical health, psychiatric comorbidity, and suicidality.

Although the negative implications of adolescent-onset MDD for functioning are well-documented, a small body of literature suggests that it is MDD recurrence, rather than early onset, that accounts for this impairment. Hammen, Brennan, Keenan-Miller, and Herr (2008) compared adolescents with MDD onset prior to age 15 who did and did not experience recurrence, on a number of psychosocial outcomes at age 20, and found that the recurrent group had more severe and pervasive impairment in relationship, school and work, financial, and physical health domains.

DD usually has an early and insidious onset in childhood, adolescence, or young adulthood (mean age 15 years) and has a chronic course. DD is termed **early-onset** if the onset of diagnostic symptoms is prior to age 21. **Late-onset** DD is rarer and is designated if the onset of diagnostic symptoms is during or after age 21. Research examining the lifetime prevalence rates of depression in US adolescents found an overall rate of 11.7% for MDD or DD, with a 15.9% rate for female and 7.7% rate for male adolescents (Merikangas et al., 2010). Early-onset depressives have higher rates of depressive personality traits and disorders than late-onset depressives and have higher rates of comorbid personality disorders (Klein et al., 1999).

MDE and MDD appear less frequently among older adults than at earlier ages (Hasin, Goodwin, Stinson, & Grant, 2005). A recent study found prevalence rates of MDD and DD in adults over 65 to be 3.1% and 0.5%, respectively (Byers, Yaffe, Covinsky, Friedman, & Bruce, 2010). This is similar to other reported rates ranging from 1% 5% in most large-scale epidemiological investigations, with the majority of studies reporting prevalence rates in the lower end of that range. There may be clear reasons for the low rates of depressive disorders in older adults, including the fact that depressed individuals die earlier. Another theory is that older adults possess psychological and social factors and capacities that appear to buffer against depression in the context of stressful events and biological risks (Hendrie et al., 2006).

> **Prevalence of MDD or DD in adults 65+ is lower than in younger adults (3.1% for MDD and 0.5% for DD)**

In contrast to young adults with DD, older adults present with late age of onset, without MDD and other psychiatric disorders, and with a low rate of family history of mood disorders. They often have stressors such as loss of social support, bereavement, and cerebrovascular or neurodegenerative pathology. A minority of older DD adults report chronic depression dating from youth, with psychiatric comorbidity similar to young adults with DD. In older versus younger adults, DD and subsyndromal depression increase disability and lead to poorer medical outcomes (Byers et al., 2010).

Rates of depression have been reported to be higher in older women than in older men, in part due to women living longer than men. There are few differences in depression prevalence in the older population by race or ethnicity, although depressive symptoms are more common among Hispanic older women than non-Hispanic whites (Swenson, Baxter, Shetterly, Scarbro, & Hamman, 2000). Rates of MDD among older adults are substantially higher in particular subsets of the older adult population, including medical outpatients (5–10%), medical inpatients (10–12%), and residents of long-term care facilities (14–42%) (Djernes, 2006).

1.3.3 Ethnicity and Cultural and Socioeconomic Differences

The WHO World Mental Health (WMH) Survey Initiative assessed a set of DSM-IV disorders in countries from every continent (Kessler & Bromet, 2013). The 12-month prevalence estimate of DSM-IV MDE in 18 countries ranged from 2.2% (Japan) to 10.4% (Brazil). The midpoint across all countries was 5%, and the weighted average 12-month prevalence was 5.5% for the 10 highest income and 5.9% for the eight low-middle income countries. The National Health and Nutrition Examination Survey III (NHANES III; Riolo, Nguyen, Greden, & King, 2005) found that the prevalence of MDD differed significantly by racial or ethnic group, with the highest prevalence in White participants (10.4%) versus Mexican Americans (8%) and African Americans (7.5%). Mexican American and White patients had significantly earlier onset of MDD compared with African Americans. Persons of any ethnicity living in poverty had nearly 1.5 times the prevalence rate of MDD. Lack of education (< 8 years of school) was significantly associated with prevalence of MDD only for Mexican Americans.

> **Poverty is a significant risk factor for MDD across racial/ethnic groups**

Race/ethnicity, sex, and education play a role in the prevalence of DD

In contrast to the comparative rates for MDD, the prevalence of DD (Riolo, Nguyen, Greden, & King, 2005) was significantly greater among African Americans (7.5%) and Mexican Americans (7.4%) compared with White Americans (5.7%). After controlling for poverty, lack of education remained a significant risk factor for DD. In addition, significant interactions occurred between race or ethnicity, sex, and education in relation to prevalence of DD. Specifically, for White respondents (of both sexes), a precipitous decline in prevalence of DD was seen with any education beyond middle school (> 8 years of education); however, for Mexican American and African American participants, the effect of education on reducing DD prevalence was only found for females.

1.4   Course and Prognosis

1.4.1   Dysthymic Disorder: Course

It is estimated that 90% of DD patients will develop an MDE in their lifetime

Most patients diagnosed with DD report an insidious onset of the disorder in mid-adolescence. "Pure" DD is relatively uncommon, with 90% of DD patients eventually developing an MDE (Klein, Shankman, & Rose, 2008). There are relatively few long-term outcome studies in the treatment of DD, and study comparisons are difficult because of varying methodologies. However, research (Klein, Shankman, & Rose, 2008) does support that a substantial proportion of sufferers do not experience a sustained recovery. Klein, Shankman, and Rose (2008) reported protracted symptoms and high relapse rates in a cohort of DD patients 5 and 10 years after diagnosis. These researchers found an estimated 5-year recovery rate from DD of 53% and determined that there was a 45% chance of relapse into another MDE. These dysthymic patients met criteria for a mood disorder a full 70% of the time during the 10-year follow-up period. During the course of the follow-up, they reported significantly more symptoms and lower functioning and were significantly more likely to attempt suicide and to be hospitalized than were patients with episodic MDE. Finally, among patients with DD who had never experienced an MDE before entry into the study, the estimated risk of having a first lifetime major depressive episode was 76.9% (Klein et al., 2008).

Almost all patients with DD will experience an exacerbation or MDE during course of disease

In their 10-year follow-up, Klein and colleagues (2008) reported that the estimated rate of recovery from DD was 73.9%, the median time to recovery was 52 months, and the estimated relapse rate was 71.4%. Although theirs was a naturalistic study, Klein et al. (2008) collected data regarding pharmacotherapy and psychotherapy in the 3 months prior to each assessment and looked at the impact on depressive symptoms. They report that greater pharmacotherapy use in the 3 months before each follow-up assessment predicted significantly greater depressive symptoms, coefficient = 0.902; SE = 0.336, $t(81)$ = 2.69, p = 0.008. Klein et al. (2008) propose that although this could indicate that pharmacotherapy had an adverse effect on course, it is more likely that patients with poorer prognoses received more pharmacotherapy. The researchers also examined levels of psychotherapy in the 3 months before each follow-up assessment and found that it did not predict depressive symptoms, coefficient = 0.421; *SE* = 0.374, *t*(81) = 1.13, *p* = .26. In light of the limited associations between treatment and course, treatment was not included as a covariate in the analyses in the study by Klein et al., and they did not attempt to use treatment to explain changes in rates. What Klein and colleagues (2008) did report is that almost all patients with DD experienced an MDE at some point during the course of their disease, thus meeting the criteria for double depression. Patients with double depression experience significantly higher levels of depression and spend more time in depressive episodes and less time fully recovered than patients with episodic MDE (Klein et al., 2008; Sansone & Sansone, 2009).

1.4.2   Major Depressive Disorder: Course

Longitudinal studies have also consistently shown MDD to be a chronic disorder, with high rates of recurrence (Rubio, Markowitz, & Alegria, 2011). For those diagnosed with MDD, the likelihood of remaining depressed for many years is high (30% are still depressed after 1 year, 20% after 2 years, 12% after 5 years) (Grant et al., 2004). Several community-based studies of MDD have shown that 20% develop a chronic course and about 30–50% have a recurrent course, and findings from a primary care setting support a similar pattern (Grant et al., 2004). The risk of recurrence after recovery is extremely high: 36% after 1 year following recovery, 40% after 2 years, 60% after 5 years, and greater than 90% after 30 years (Keller, 2013). As many as 57% of patients diagnosed with MDD at baseline had not recovered after 39 months, which is consistent with findings from a study in primary care, where 53% of the adult population diagnosed with MDD at baseline had not recovered after 3.5 years (Stegenga, Kamphuis, Nazareth, & Geerlings, 2012).

MDD has high rates of recurrence and chronicity

1.4.3   Onset Age

There are several important differences in the characteristics and course of early- versus late-onset DD patients. Compared with late-onset patients, early-onset patients seek treatment more often and report significantly higher rates of lifetime MDEs and comorbid Axis I and II disorders (Sansone & Sansone, 2009). They use emotional coping styles more than other strategies and they report greater stress responsivity, more frequent familial mood disorders, and higher rates of childhood adversity (McCullough et al., 1990). Patients who have their onset of MDD before adulthood appear to have a particularly severe and chronic condition. They are more likely to be female, have a longer duration of the disorder, longer and more numerous episodes, greater symptom severity, increased suicidality, and more comorbidities and atypical symptoms (Klein & Santiago, 2003).

Early- vs. late-onset DD patients appear to have a more severe and chronic depressive symptoms

1.4.4   Impact of Treatment on Clinical Course

Only 28–50% of people diagnosed with PDD will receive treatment

Only 28–50% of patients with PDD receive some form of treatment, which is unfortunate because PDD very rarely spontaneously remits (Al-Harbi, 2012). PDD often develops over years and is likely to persist unless treatment is initiated and outcomes are monitored to ensure that treatment response is achieved and sustained. Treatment is typically a combination of pharmacotherapy and psychotherapy, and may also include electroconvulsive therapy (ECT) or transcranial magnetic stimulation (TMS). Of those who do receive treatment, studies have found that 60–70% of patients with DD and MDD will benefit substantially from treatment (Rush et al., 2006). Unfortunately, a significant number of patients remain very depressed even after multiple aggressive treatments. According to the Sequenced Treatment Alternatives to Relieve Depression (STAR*D) study, 50–66% of patients with depression do not recover fully on an antidepressant medication, while 33% of patients achieve remission (Warden, Rush, Trivedi, Fava, & Wisniewski, 2007). Patients with DD may take longer to respond to pharmacotherapy and need higher doses of pharmacotherapy to reach remission of symptoms. Interestingly, early-onset in MDD does not appear to be associated with poorer response to pharmacotherapy treatment (Zisook et al., 2007).

60–70% of patients will benefit from treatment

50–66% of patients will not recover fully on an antidepressant

10–30% of people with PDD will not respond to any treatment

Of those patients who do not respond to treatment, 10–30% exhibit ongoing symptoms coupled with difficulties in social and occupational function, poor physical health, suicidal thoughts, and increased health care utilization (Al-Harbi, 2012). MDD that demonstrates a poor or unsatisfactory response to two adequate (optimal dosage and duration) trials of two different classes of antidepressants has been proposed as an operational definition of treatment-resistant depression (TRD). Unfortunately, approximately 30% of patients with TRD do not respond to any treatment (Al-Harbi, 2012).

1.5   Differential Diagnosis

PDD is often insidious and may be confused with other mood or personality disorders. A number of other psychiatric and physical conditions can mimic PDD symptoms. Some of the most common differential diagnoses are presented in Table 2, along with characteristics that differentiate these disorders from PDD.

The most obvious differential diagnosis for PDD is an acute depressive disorder such as an MDE, adjustment disorder with depressed mood, or grief. Severity, duration, or number of depressive symptoms typically differentiate reactive and acute depressive disorders from PDD. Generally speaking, the duration and severity of depressive symptoms is less in patients who meet criteria for an adjustment disorder or who are experiencing grief. Patients may meet criteria for a single MDE and not meet criteria for PDD – in fact, such patients would presumably have more numerous and perhaps more severe depressive symptoms than those diagnosed with DD, but of a shorter duration.

Criteria for generalized anxiety disorder (GAD) state that the diagnosis should not be made if the worry occurs only during an episode of depression.

Table 2
Characteristics of PDD Versus Other Mood Disorders

Disorder	Difference from PDD
Adjustment disorder	Symptoms occur in response to stressor; lack of chronicity; less severe
Bipolar disorders	Manic or hypomanic symptoms are present or have been in the past
Disruptive mood dysregulation disorder	Symptoms of temper outbursts manifested verbally or behaviorally
Due to medical conditions	Symptoms attributable to direct pathophysiology effects of medical condition
Other specified depressive disorder	Full criteria for other mood disorder not met, but significant symptoms present
Psychotic disorders	Not diagnosed as PDD if depressive symptoms occur only when psychotic
Premenstrual dysphoric disorder	Symptoms are attributable to menstrual cycle changes
Single MDE(s)	Lack of chronicity; 2-week duration of symptoms versus 1- to 2-year duration
Substance/medication induced	Symptoms attributable to substance, medication, or toxin

Note. MDE = major depressive episode; PDD = persistent depressive disorder.

However, if GAD occurs first, both diagnoses may apply. Since the hallmarks of PDD are avoidant behavior, social withdraw, and lack of interest in others, it may be challenging to make a differential diagnosis between PDD and GAD, social phobia, or avoidant personality disorder. In such cases, the anxiety diagnoses must have been established prior to PDD for both diagnoses to be given.

Sleep difficulties are a classic symptom of PDD and other depressive disorders but may also be related to anxiety disorders or a primary sleep disorder. If insomnia or hypersomnolence is a presenting complaint, it is necessary for the clinician to conduct a thorough investigation of the symptoms to determine if the sleep difficulties are primary symptoms of insomnia, or another sleep disorder, or related to a mood or anxiety disorder.

Differentiating personality disorders from PDD can be challenging. Depressive personality disorder is no longer in the DSM-5 but was described in previous versions as a pervasive pattern of depressive cognitions and behaviors that occurs across situations. The essential features of a personality disorder are impairments in personality (self and interpersonal) functioning and the presence of pathological personality traits, which may or may not be present in PDD. Patients may have overlapping symptoms and meet criteria for a personality disorder and PDD, in which case both would be diagnosed.

Differentiating personality disorders from PDD can be challenging

Depressive personality disorder is no longer in the DSM-5

1.6   Comorbidities

PDD can be comorbid with any other psychiatric or medical disorder, and it has been estimated that the vast majority (up to 75%) of DD patients suffer from some comorbid psychiatric disorder and have higher rates of physical illnesses (Blanco et al., 2010). Anxiety disorders are frequently comorbid in patients with PDD (approximately 50% of those diagnosed with DD), and the disorders share many symptoms (Thase, Friedman, & Howland, 2001). Typical comorbid anxiety disorders include panic disorder, simple phobia, GAD, and social phobia. Depressed patients with comorbid anxiety are more severely depressed and are found to be at a greater risk for suicide and to have greater functional impairment (Kornstein & Schneider, 2001; Thase, Friedman, & Howland, 2001). If both an anxiety disorder and PDD criteria are met, both should be diagnosed.

> **Anxiety disorders are frequently comorbid in patients with PDD and the disorders share many symptoms**

Early-onset PDD has been strongly associated with comorbid personality disorders. The prevalence of personality disorders in PDD can range from 14% to 85% with a mean of about 50% (Kornstein & Schneider, 2001). Early-onset PDD is specifically strongly associated with DSM-IV Cluster B and C personality disorders. Many of the personality disorders share signs, symptoms, and characteristics of PDD, including feelings of sadness, hopelessness, despair, poor functioning, and early developmental trauma or loss (Kornstein & Schneider, 2001).

> **Early-onset DD is frequently comorbid with personality disorders**

Patients with somatoform disorders, such as hypochondriasis and somatization, have increased rates of PDD, and patients with PDD endorse symptoms of pain at high rates (an average of 65% comorbidity rate) (Bair, Robinson, Katon, & Kroenke, 2003). Substance use disorders are frequently comorbid with PDD, and alcohol dependence is especially common among those diagnosed with PDD. The comorbidity rates between alcohol dependence and MDD and DD were 11.03% and 9.62%, respectively (Grant et al., 2004). PDD is consistently associated with poor health, including more specific health conditions such as chronic fatigue, migraine headaches, high blood pressure, arthritis, and back pain. DD patients may also experience low quality of life, disability, poor social support, marital issues, and negative responses to stress (Satyanarayana, Enns, Cox, & Sareen, 2009).

> **Substance use disorders, especially alcohol use disorders, frequently co-occur with PDD**

1.7   Diagnostic Procedures and Documentation

Making an accurate diagnosis of PDD is important because chronicity has been found to significantly impact patients' responses to treatment, with chronic patients taking longer to respond to pharmacotherapy, demonstrating higher nonresponse rates, and exhibiting greater recurrence and relapse rates than patients with episodic MDEs (Keller, 1990). Failure to diagnose the chronicity of the depressive disorder may result in inadequate treatment (McCullough, 2012a). As McCullough states: "In missing the early roots of the patient's dilemma, psychotherapy fails because clinicians do not address the disastrous and crippling early developmental experiences" (McCullough, 2012a, p. 9). Accurate diagnosis is made challenging by the complexity of unipolar depression diagnoses and the serious developmental limitations of the PDD patient, which may lead to the clinician's overestimate of the patient's abilities (McCullough, 2000). Clinicians can also easily miss the onset of depressive symptoms and administer treatment based only on current symptoms, which could lead to ineffective treatment and lack of therapeutic response.

There are multiple tools to diagnose and determine the severity level and functional impairment of depression over time. In the following sections, I focus on commonly used and well-supported measures to diagnose PDD that are also relatively easy to access and convenient to administer. I have not included all available assessment tools. You may have measures that are preferable for use in your own practice.

1.7.1   Diagnostic Interviews

There are a number of diagnostic interviews used to diagnosis DD and MDD, which are also used to diagnose PDD. Most of these were developed by researchers to assess the relevant DSM criteria at the time, and many have been revised to reflect the DSM-5 criteria. The goals of a diagnostic interview for PDD include differentiating PDD from other symptoms and disorders, and establishing whether there is a persistent course of depression versus an acute or episodic depressive disorder. Clinician evaluation helps to achieve clarity in diagnosis and determine which psychotherapeutic approach may be most appropriate. In patients with late-onset depression who do not have antecedent early-onset dysthymia, the onset of depressive symptoms often begins during their mid-20s and is preceded by some crisis or significant stress event (McCullough et al., 1996). Early-onset DD is important to identify because it is often associated with a developmental history of abuse or maltreatment (Uher, 2011), which may impact the choice and duration of treatment.

Early versions of diagnostic interviews listed criteria for disorders, and eventually researchers developed standardized questions to ascertain results for each criterion. One of the first was the published set of questions in the Research Diagnostic Criteria (RDC; Spitzer, Endicott, & Robins, 1975), which became the **Schedule for Affective Disorders and Schizophrenia** (SADS; Spitzer, Endicott, & Robins, 1978). The SADS has versions that assess lifetime (SADS-L), current diagnoses, and changes in diagnosis (SADS-C), and there is a version for children and their parents (Kiddie-SADS; Chambers et al., 1985). The SADS has been largely replaced by other structured interviews that follow diagnostic criteria such as those of the DSM-IV and DSM-5. Standardizing questions for diagnosis in this fashion was crucial in improving the reliability of diagnoses.

Structured diagnostic interviews use standardized questions to determine criteria for DSM disorders

For practicing clinicians, I recommend the **Structured Clinical Interview for the DSM-5** (SCID-5; APA, 2013), the **Mini International Neuropsychiatric Interview-5** (MINI-5; Sheehan, 2015), and the **Diagnostic Interview for Anxiety, Mood, and OCD and Related Neuropsychiatric Disorders** (DIAMOND; Tolin et al., 2016), with the choice based ultimately on the training, time limits, and preferences of the administering clinician. These interviews have all been updated for the newest version of the DSM, but psychometric data regarding DSM-5 versions have not been published for all of them.

The **SCID** has a clinical version published by the APA and is constructed in modules for different sets of diagnoses, with sequences of questions and decision points. A clinician or trained mental health professional familiar with the DSM classification and diagnostic criteria administers the SCID. The reliability of the procedure is well established, with kappas of 0.81 for DD (Lobbestael, Leurgans, & Arntz, 2011) and 0.80 for MDD (Zanarini et al., 2000) for the SCID-IV, but there are as yet no psychometric data published for the SCID-5. The validity of the SCID is hard to establish due to the fact that validity is generally measured by determining the agreement between diagnosis made by the assessment and a **gold standard**. However, such a gold standard for psychiatric diagnosis remains elusive, and in fact, the SCID has been used as the gold standard (Shear et al., 2000). The SCID can take up to 2 hrs to administer, especially in patients with multiple disorders or those who do not express themselves clearly or succinctly.

The **MINI-5** (Sheehan, 2015) was designed to be an even shorter structured interview and was developed jointly by psychiatrists and clinicians in the US and Europe to meet DSM and ICD criteria. With an administration time of approximately 15 min, it was designed to meet the need for a short but accurate structured psychiatric interview for multicenter clinical trials and epidemiology studies and to be used as a first step in outcome tracking in nonresearch clinical settings. There are several versions, including: the MINI-Screen, the MINI-Plus, and the MINI-Kid. The reliability of the MINI-IV, for which the most recent data are available, is strong, with reported kappas of 0.84 for MDD and 0.52 for DD, when compared with the SCID (Sheehan et al., 1998). Specificities and negative predictive values ranged from 0.97 to 0.99, with positive predictive values of 87% for MDD and 45% for DD (Sheehan et al., 1998). A disadvantage of the MINI-5 is that it does not assess for PDD specifically, and to date, no psychometric data have been published for the MINI-5.

The **DIAMOND** (Tolin et al., 2016) is a semistructured interview that targets the diagnostic criteria for a range of DSM-5 disorders. It takes about an hour to administer. The DIAMOND diagnoses demonstrate very good to excellent inter-rater reliability, with kappas of 0.62 to 1.00, and good to excellent test–retest reliability using cutoff criteria from the DSM-5 field trials with kappas of 0.59 to 1.00 (Tolin et al., 2016). Comparison to a gold standard for DSM-5 is not possible, since there has been no psychometric data yet published for the SCID-5 (First et al., 2015) or the MINI-5 (Sheehan, 2015). Overall, the DIAMOND appears ideal due to its convenient length and reportedly strong reliability and the fact that it was specifically constructed using the DSM-5 field trial criteria and cutoffs (Tolin et al., 2016).

Making a diagnosis based on a diagnostic interview can be challenging with PDD patients precisely because of the chronicity of disease and insidious and uneven progression of symptoms and severity. Knowledge of the onset, severity, and duration of symptoms is important in differentiating forms of PDD from nonchronic depression and from each other. In recent years, clinical course methodology has received increasing emphasis in the diagnosis of mood disorders. A timeline formulation can be used in addition to a diagnostic interview when making the diagnosis of PDD. McCullough, Clark, Klein,

---

SCID-IV has good reliability and is considered the gold standard by some

No psychometric data are available for the SCID-5

The MINI takes about 15 min to administer

MINI-IV has good reliability and validity, but no psychometric data are available yet for MINI-5

Mapping clinical course and psychosocial functioning with timeline method can be helpful in PDD diagnosis

and First (2016b) developed a **Timeline Course Graphing Scale (TCGS) for the DSM-5 mood disorders** to aid in the diagnosis of patients with PDD. The scale is used during the diagnostic interview in an iterative process with the patient, and involves drawing a mood timeline to illustrate the clinical course of the disorder over time. Clinicians administering this scale use the DSM-5 diagnostic criteria to discriminate between moods and severity levels of elevated or depressed moods along the timeline. Diagnosis begins in the present moment, and the clinician works backward in time with the patient to assess changes in mood over time. Techniques of helping the patient recall past moods are similar to those used in a Timeline Followback (TLFB; Sobell & Sobell, 2000) procedure, in which prompts about important dates, such as holidays, are used to help aid the patient's memories when judging symptom occurrence or severity.

McCullough et al. (2016a) also developed a procedure to graph the quality of psychosocial functioning affected by symptom severity. This clinical course graphing scale is similar to the TCGS, with severity of functional impact assessed on the perpendicular axis and clinical timeline on the horizontal axis. Functional impairment of psychosocial functioning is rated on a scale from 0 (*no interference*) to 10 (*severe interference*). Lyketsos and colleagues (Lyketsos, Nestadt, Cwi, Heithof, & Eaton, 1994) also recommend a life chart interview to assess the course of depression.

TCGS is used to chart the quality of psychosocial functioning affected by symptom severity

1.7.2　Clinician Rating Scales

Clinician rating scales assess one or more dimensions of depression as continuous variables, and they are used to assess symptoms over time. Use of these scales assumes that the rater is trained and experienced. Below are a few selected rating scales that I find most useful.

Clinician rating scales can be used to assess severity of symptoms and to evaluate change over time

The **Hamilton Depression Rating Scale** (HDRS; Hamilton, 1960) is a well-known instrument that is frequently used in pharmacotherapy trials for depression. It is a rational scale designed for use with patients already diagnosed with depression. The HDRS was originally designed to be completed by two raters who would sum their results, but this is typically not done currently. The original scale consisted of 21 items, although only 17 were counted for the score. Each item was rated on a 3- or 5-point scale. There is now a 24-item version of the scale, which includes three cognitive symptoms added to the original scale. The HDRS covers all of the DSM-5 criteria for PDD. Different researchers have used different cutoffs, but generally a cutoff of between 7 and 10 is used to define who is no longer depressed, with lower scores associated with fewer symptoms. Scores above 25 are considered severe (Hamilton, 1960). Scoring criteria can be found in Table 3. Assessment time is typically about 20 min. Inter-rater reliabilities generally have been good, as has been concurrent validity, and the sensitivity is reported to be 86.4% and specificity 92.2% (Strik, Honig, Lousberg, & Denollet, 2001). However, recently some researchers have proposed that the HDRS is psychometrically and conceptually flawed beyond repair and have advocated discontinuing its use in favor of more current assessments (Bagby, Ryder, Schuller, & Marshall, 2004).

Table 3
Scoring Criteria for the Hamilton Depression Rating Scale

Score	Severity
0–7	Minimal depression
8–13	Mild depression
14–19	Moderate depression
20–25	Severe depression
> 25	Very severe depression

HDRS and MADRS are two commonly used clinician-administered rating scales for depression

A more psychometrically sound depression assessment scale is the **Montgomery–Asberg Depression Rating Scale** (MADRS; Montgomery & Asberg, 1979), which was developed specifically to determine symptom changes in clinical trials. There are 10 items on the scale, each rated on 7-point scale from 0 (*absent*) to 6 (*severe*). The overall score ranges from 0 to 60. Typical cutoff points are provided in Table 4. A self-rated version of the MADRS called the MADRS-S, which has nine questions and an overall scoring rage from 0 to 54, is often used in clinical practice and correlates reasonably well with the clinician-administered MADRS. Assessment time for the clinician-administered MADRS is typically about 20 to 60 min. The MADRS has reported concurrent validity determined by correlating scores with the Cornell Scale for Depression (range r = 0.74–0.93, p < .0001). The MADRS was compared with the HDRS on clinical assessments of severity of depression, and the correlation for the MADRS was 0.71, which is slightly higher than the 0.65 for the HDRS (McDowell, 2006). The authors reported inter-rater reliability that ranged from 0.89 to 0.97 for various combinations of raters in small samples of 12 to 30 patients. Intraclass coefficients for the MADRS fell between 0.66 and 0.82 (Montgomery & Asberg, 1979).

Table 4
Scoring Criteria for the Montgomery–Asberg Depression Rating Scale

Score	Severity
0–6	Normal or symptom absent
7–19	Mild depression
20–34	Moderate depression
> 34	Severe depression

Self-report scales are completed by patient to assess symptoms and severity and change in symptoms over time

1.7.3   Self-Report Scales

Self-report scales are measures that patients being assessed for depression complete on their own. These assessments can be used to screen for depression or to rate the severity of symptoms. Below are some readily available and well-accepted self-report scales used with DD, MDE and MDD, and now PDD.

The **Beck Depression Inventory** (BDI) is a popular self-assessment that has been revised into a 21-item version called the BDI-II (Beck, Steer, & Brown, 1996). Nineteen items are scored from 0 to 3, with 3 being most severe; two questions have answers regarding symptoms that can deviate from normal either by increasing or decreasing (e.g., too much sleep or too little sleep). Although all diagnostic symptoms of depression are covered, the content focuses on cognitive items, which is not surprising, given Beck's cognitive conception of depression. The BDI-II provides scoring guidelines for interpretation that can be found in Table 5. The BDI is currently available in the original format, the BDI-II, and the BDI-C (a shorter version for use in primary care offices), and it is available in 17 languages. A review (Wang & Gorenstein, 2013) found internal consistency for the BDI-II of 0.9 and test retest reliability ranging from 0.73 to 0.96. These researchers further reported a sensitivity of ≥ 0.70 and the significant diagnostic accuracy, as expressed by the area under the receiver operating characteristic curve, was around 75% and higher. Wang and Gorenstein (2013) concluded that the BDI-II is a relevant psychometric instrument, showing high reliability, capacity to discriminate between depressed and nondepressed subjects, and improved concurrent, content, and structural validity.

Table 5
Scoring Criteria for the 21-Item Beck Depression Inventory

Score	Severity
0–13	Minimal depression
14–19	Mild depression
20–28	Moderate depression
29–63	Severe depression

The **Zung Self-Rating Depression Scale** (Zung, 1974) was developed to assess factors common to depressed patients and is frequently used in pharmacotherapy trials. The scale has 20 items, with half written in a positive direction and half in a negative direction. Each question is scored on a scale from 1 (*a little*) to 4 (*most of the time*). Scores are calculated as a percentage index with the cutoff scores displayed in Table 6. Reliability of the Zung is good with a split-half reliability of 0.73 and an Cronbach's α coefficient of .82; the correlation with physician global ratings of depression was .69 (Lee, 1990).

The **Major Depression Inventory** (MDI) is a self-report mood questionnaire developed by the WHO (Bech, Rasmussen, Olsen, Noerholm, & Abildgaard, 2001). The MDI differs from other self-report inventories in that it is able to generate an ICD or DSM diagnosis of depression in addition to an estimate of symptom severity. Ten items are scored to determine symptom severity, ranging from mild, moderate, severe, to major. As a diagnostic tool, the 10 items are dichotomized for the *presence* (1) or *absence* (0) of each

Table 6
Scoring Criteria for the Zung Self-Rating Depression Scale

Score	Severity
< 50	Normal range
50–59	Minimal to mild depression
60–69	Moderate depression
70–79	Severe depression

symptom. For the diagnosis of MDD, either Item 1 or 2 should be among the five of nine items endorsed. Items 4 and 5 are combined, with only the highest answer category considered and a total number of nine items. As a measuring tool, the items are given a value (0–5) and summed up to a theoretical score of 0 to 50. The cutoff score is 26 for the diagnosis of major (moderate to severe) depression. Scoring can be found in Table 7. The sensitivity of the MDI algorithms is between 86% and 92%, while the specificity is reported to be between 82% and 86% (Bech et al., 2001).

Table 7
Scoring Criteria for the Major Depression Inventory

Score	Severity
0–20	No or doubtful depression
21–25	Mild depression
26–30	Moderate depression
31–50	Severe depression

The **Inventory of Depressive Symptomatology, Clinician Rating** (IDS-C), Self-Report (IDS-SR), Quick Inventory of Depressive Symptomatology (QIDS), Clinician Rating (QIDS-C), and Self-Report (QIDS-SR) are similar forms. The 16-item QIDS (an abbreviated version of the 30-item IDS) is designed to assess the severity of depressive symptoms. These assessments can be used to screen for depression, although they have been used predominantly as measures of symptom severity. The QIDS is easy to administer in either the clinician-rated (QIDS-C16) or patient self-report (QIDS-SR16) versions and requires minimal training (Rush et al., 2003). The QIDS-SR has good internal consistency, with Cronbach's α = .86 (Rush et al., 2003). A recent large meta-analysis (Reilly, MacGillivray, Reid, & Cameron, 2015) found a Cronbach's alpha ranging from .69 to .89 for the QIDS-SR and .65 to .87 for the QIDS-C. No studies could be found that reported test–retest reliability of either the QIDS-SR or the QIDS-C. Both versions are sensitive to change due to medications, psychotherapy, or somatic treatments, making them useful for research and clinical purposes (Reilly, MacGillivray, Reid, &

Table 8
Scoring Criteria for the Quick Inventory of Depressive Symptomatology Self-Report

Score	Severity
1–5	No depression
6–10	Mild depression
11–15	Moderate depression
16–20	Severe depression
21–27	Very severe depression

Cameron, 2015). The psychometric properties of the QIDS-SR are comparable to those of the HDRS in detecting symptom change in MDD (Reilly et al., 2015; Rush et al., 2003). Scoring cutoffs can be found in Table 8.

The **Patient Health Questionnaire-9** (PHQ-9; Spitzer, Kroenke, Williams, & Patient Health Questionnaire Study Group, 1999) is a self-reported, nine-question version of the Primary Care Evaluation of Mental Disorders. The Patient Health Questionnaire-2 (PHQ-2) is a shorter version of the PHQ-9, with two screening questions to assess the presence of a depressed mood and a loss of interest or pleasure in routine activities; a positive response to either question indicates further testing is required. The PHQ-9 establishes the clinical diagnosis of depression and can be used to track the severity of symptoms over time (Kroenke, Spitzer, & Williams, 2001). The cutoff of the PHQ-9 is > 10, and the scale has a sensitivity of 88% and a specificity of 88% for major depression. See Table 9 for scoring criteria. The internal reliability of the PHQ-9 is excellent, with Cronbach's alpha ranging from .86 to .89 (Kroenke, Spitzer, & Williams, 2001). The correlation between the PHQ-9 completed by the patient and that administered telephonically within 48 hrs was .84, and the mean scores were nearly identical (5.08 vs. 5.03) (Kroenke, Spitzer, & Williams, 2001).

Table 9
Scoring Criteria for the Patient Health Questionnaire-9

Score	Severity
0–4	Minimal
5–9	Mild depression
10–14	Moderate depression
15–19	Moderately severe depression
20–27	Severe depression

1.7.4   Scales Assessing Constructs Related to PDD

Additional scales to assess constructs related to PDD evaluate the underlying constructs of theories of PDD. These typically revolve around behaviors, cognitions, and functional status, including coping, stress, and interpersonal functioning. Such assessments are typically not used to make a diagnosis or determine severity of the disorder, but instead are assumed to be important components of the etiology and/or impact of the diagnosis. They may also relate to the theorized causes of depression or mechanisms of action of the proposed treatment or therapy.

Behavioral assessments can evaluate depressed behaviors as well as lack of reinforcing behaviors

Behavioral assessments can include direct observation of behavior or coding of such, but these methodologies have not been standardized. Assessments such as the Pleasant Events Schedule and Unpleasant Events Schedule (Lewinsohn & Talkington, 1979; MacPhillamy & Lewinsohn, 1982) have been used to evaluate the amount of reinforcing and punishing behaviors in a depressed person's daily life. Self-control skills such as the Self-Control Questionnaire for Depression (Fuchs & Rehm, 1977) may be conceptualized as part of this cluster of behaviorally related assessments.

Negative thoughts, beliefs, and attitudes can be used to assess depression

Cognitive assessments include the Beck Hopelessness Scale (BHS; Beck, Weissman, Lester, & Trexler, 1974), a 20-item self-report inventory that was designed to measure three major aspects of hopelessness: feelings about the future, loss of motivation, and expectations. The BHS measures the extent of the respondent's negative attitudes, or pessimism, about the future and is used as an indicator of suicidal risk in depressed people who have made suicide attempts. The Attributional Style Questionnaire (ASQ; Peterson, Semmel, von Baeyer, & Seligman, 1982) was developed from Seligman's learned helplessness theory of depression and assumes that a psychological vulnerability to depression is based in part on a patient's inferences about the causes of positive and negative events. The Automatic Thoughts Questionnaire (ATQ; Hollon & Kendall, 1980) assesses negative and positive self-statements. Negative self-statements are associated with increased vulnerability in the cognitive theory of depression. The Dysfunctional Attitudes Scale (DAS; Weissman & Beck, 1978) is similar to the ATQ in that it assesses maladaptive negative thoughts and assumptions.

Stress and functioning can be used in the assessment of depression

Assessments related to perceived functioning, quality of life, and stress are too numerous to detail. I list below some of the measures I find useful. The Perceived Stress Scale (PSS; Cohen, Kamarck, & Mermelstein, 1983) is one of the most widely used psychological instruments for measuring the perception of stress. The Brief Symptom Inventory (BSI; Derogatis, 1993) evaluates psychological distress. The Quality of Life Scale (Flanagan, 1982) is a valid instrument for measuring quality of life across patient groups and cultures and is conceptually distinct from health status or other causal indicators of quality of life. The COPE Inventory (Carver, Scheier, & Weintraub, 1989) is used to assess a broad range of coping responses, several of which have an explicit basis in theory. The Ways of Coping Questionnaire (Folkman & Lazarus, 1988) also identifies the processes people use in coping with stressful situations.

Additional tools to explore interpersonal functioning and attachment include the Social Adjustment Scale (SAS; Weissman & Bothwell, 1976), which assesses social skills and was developed to be used with **interpersonal psychotherapy** (IPT). The **interpersonal circle** (IPC) or circumplex is a model for assessing interpersonal dispositions. Two orthogonal axes define the IPC: a vertical axis of dominance, control, or agency, and a horizontal axis of friendliness, warmth, or communion. Inventories designed to measure interpersonal dispositions from every IPC region typically divide the IPC into eight or more octants. As one moves around the circle, each octant reflects a progressive blend of the two axial dimensions. The Impact Message Inventory (IMI; Kiesler & Schmidt, 2006) is a self-report inventory designed to measure internal interpersonal reactions, referred to as **impact messages**. It is used in both IPT and the **cognitive behavioral analysis system of psychotherapy** (CBASP). The Adult Attachment Inventory (AAI; Main, Goldwyn, & Hesse, 2002) is a procedure for assessing attachment in adults and is often used in patients with trauma histories.

It may be useful to assess interpersonal functioning, impact, values, or desired functioning of PDD patients

2

Theories and Models of Persistent Depressive Disorders

Biopsychosocial model attributes disease to interaction of biological, psychological, and social factors

The etiology of PDD can be conceptualized within a multifactorial biopsychosocial framework. The biopsychosocial model attributes disease outcome to the variable interactions of biological factors (genetic, biochemical, biological), psychological factors (mood, personality, behavior), and social factors (cultural, familial, socioeconomic). Accompanying this framework is a **diathesis–stress model**, which has been increasingly popular in describing the etiology of PDD. The diathesis–stress model explains a disorder as the result of an interaction between a predisposed vulnerability and current psychosocial stress. The influences within such a model include genetic and biological factors, developmental and learning history, social and cultural influences, coping strategies, personality, chronic stress, trauma, and medical illness. Although there are multiple theories and models used to explain the development and continuation of depression, less research has been conducted specifically for PDD. Current major theories or models of depression will be reviewed here, with a focus on PDD and models that have associated empirically supported treatment approaches for PDD.

Diathesis–stress views disorders as interaction between a genetic vulnerability and psychosocial stress

2.1   Biological Models

There is a strong biological component to PDD

All forms of PDD are thought to have strong biological components in their etiology. Depression has been associated with multiple neurochemical changes, including deficiencies in norepinephrine, serotonin, and dopamine, and to variations of dopamine autoreceptors, 5-GT receptors, alpha-NE or beta-NE receptors. These changes may also be influenced by hormonal variations that contribute to the vast array of individual differences biologically and symptom-wise within and across depressed patients. In addition, chronic stress or trauma can provoke, exacerbate, or help maintain MDD, DD, and PDD.

2.1.1   Genetics

There is a genetic component to MDD and DD; depression runs in families

It is fairly well established that there is a genetic component of depression and that depression runs in families (Howland & Thase, 1991). Prevalence rates of MDD, DD, and double depression differ in families, suggesting their distinctions, even though they have substantial similarities. Environmental stress may be a greater influence in the etiology of DD, less severe depression, or early-onset depression than in the etiology of MDD, and the genetic contribution appears to be greater for more severe, recurrent, melancholic, or psychotic depression (Griffiths, Ravindran, Merali, & Anisman, 2000).

Scientists have not found a specific gene or series of genes that cause depression, but have found certain variations in genes, called polymorphisms, that may increase the risk for depression. Genes and their variations are important because they help control the metabolism of neurotransmitters and their receptors, and they control the numbers of particular types of neurons and their synaptic connections, the intracellular transduction of neuronal signals, and the speed with which all of these can change in response to environmental stressors (Lohoff, 2010).

No specific gene has been found for depression, but gene variations (polymorphisms), may increase risk

2.1.2   Monoamine Hypothesis

The **monoaminergic systems** (serotonin, norepinephrine, and dopamine) have received the most attention in the neurobiology of MDD, and most classes of antidepressants target these monoaminergic systems. Investigation into the neurobiology of depression has especially focused on serotonin and norepinephrine (Lohoff, 2010). An enzyme called **monoamine oxidase** is involved in removing serotonin and dopamine from the brain. The monoamine hypothesis posits that depressed patients have low levels of these neurotransmitters and that antidepressant medications that increase the levels help improve depressive symptoms. We know that unfortunately this does not happen for every patient. Additionally, research has demonstrated that lowering serotonin levels does not induce depression in all people (Cools et al., 2005). Overall, there appear to be several factors that contribute to a patient's vulnerability to the effects of lowered serotonin on depressive symptoms. There is evidence for biological differences within chronically depressed patients, with strong support for a greater monoamine oxidase imbalance in early-onset DD versus late-onset DD (Versiani, Amrein, Stabl, & International Collaborative Study Group, 1997).

The monoamine hypothesis posits that depressed patients have low levels of these neurotransmitters s

2.1.3   Serotonin

The **serotonin transporter gene** is the most studied with respect to PDD because it has a polymorphism (a "short" vs. "long" allele) that appears to slow down the synthesis of the serotonin transporter (Jans, Riedel, Markus, & Blokland, 2007). This reduces the speed with which serotonin neurons can adapt to changes in their stimulation. This polymorphism may influence a person's sensitivity to stress, thus increasing vulnerability to depression. This is a good example of the diathesis–stress model of disease. In this case, stress is a precipitating factor for depression in patients with genetic vulnerabilities. Stress interacts with a patient's genetic makeup to influence risk for developing PDD. Research to support this can be found in birth cohort studies. Specifically, Caspi et al. (2003) conducted a prospective study with a cohort of patients born around the same time (same birth cohort). They found that in their cohort, having a MDD in the past year was best predicted by the combination of

Polymorphisms in serotonin transporter gene may interact with stress to increase vulnerability to depression

having the short allele (polymorphism) of the serotonin transporter gene and having had multiple stressful life events in the past 5 years. Such interactive findings have been consistently reported, and the effects of multiple genes and psychosocial stress on depression are only starting to be explored.

2.1.4   Dopamine

Dopamine is increasingly thought to play an important role in the pathophysiology of MDD. Perceived threats or stress trigger the amygdala to increase levels of dopamine in the prefrontal cortex and the ventral striatum. Inhibitory feedback creates a return to homeostasis, but stress can disrupt the feedback system by alerting striatal levels of brain-derived neurotrophic factor. This abnormal feedback in patients with depression may reduce striatal dopamine causing additional anhedonia or other depressive symptoms such as the tendency to attribute inappropriate salience to even mildly negative stimuli (McClung & Nestler, 2008). In fact, a polymorphism in the dopamine type 2 receptor gene has been found to influence the effect of past stressful life events on current depressive mood (Elovainio et al., 2007). Again, we see a diathesis–stress model in action, with the dopamine system potentially influencing vulnerability to MDD via interaction with stress in the current environment of the individual.

> **Dopamine polymorphisms may influence the effect past stress can have on worsening depression**

2.1.5   Brain-Derived Neurotrophic Factor

Another polymorphism that may moderate the interactive effect of the serotonin transporter and stress is located on the gene that codes for **brain-derived neurotrophic factor**. This is a growth factor that has an important role in the genesis, development, and survival of brain cells. A common polymorphism in this gene ("Val" vs. "Met") affects intracellular transport and secretion of brain-derived neurotrophic factor, impacting the hippocampus size and functioning, leading to hippocampal hypersensitivity to stress (Bath & Lee, 2006) and ultimately depression. There also appears to be an additive effect of having the short allele of the serotonin transporter, the Met allele and psychosocial stress, with an increased risk of depression resulting from having all three, even if the stress took place in childhood. Further evidence for a role of brain-derived neurotrophic factor in the pathophysiology of MDD comes from postmortem studies, which have found low levels of brain-derived neurotrophic factor in the hippocampus and prefrontal cortex of symptomatic depressed patients (Martinowich, Manji, & Lu, 2007).

> **Genetic polymorphisms may interact with psychosocial stress to increase risk for PDD**

2.1.6   Neuroendocrine Models

In studies of the impact of psychosocial adversity during childhood on the risk of adult depression, it is often difficult to separate the effects of genes from those of the environment. This is because in the early environment, the same genetics are often at work in parents and children (e.g., when they are biologically related), informing behaviors of both. Thus, studies with nonhumans are used to help us understand the interaction of genes and stress. For example, monkeys temporarily reared by peers rather than by their mothers develop exaggerated stress responses associated with abnormalities in serotonin activity as well as in the hypothalamic-pituitary-adrenal axis. Data from studies in rats also suggest that early developmental experiences can alter the reactivity of the hypothalamic-pituitary-adrenal axis. These studies have demonstrated that these alterations are at least partially mediated by modifications in genes that do not involve any actual changes in the underlying DNA (epigenetic changes) (Tsankova, Renthal, Kumar, & Nestler, 2007). Specifically, the hippocampi of adult rats deprived of maternal care during infancy display epigenetic modifications in the gene for the glucocorticoid receptor, and this modification mediates the effects of cortisol released from the adrenal glands in response to stress. The process that leads to epigenetic changes, which affect gene transcription, is impacted by serotonin. The resulting changes in glucocorticoid receptor expression in the hippocampus increase the reactivity of the hypothalamic- pituitary-adrenal axis. This epigenetic process may even occur in utero and is thought to be extremely long lasting. This might help explain why people with MDD often show abnormalities in this neuroendocrine system. Work in the area of DD also suggests that DD may stem from disturbances of neuroendocrine and neurotransmitter functioning (Griffiths, Ravindran, Merali, & Anisman, 2000).

Abnormalities in the hypothalamic-pituitary-adrenal axis are associated with MDD

A combined dysregulation of the hypothalamic and extrahypothalamic corticotropin-releasing factor systems may help explain why patients with MDD have high levels of corticotropin-releasing factor and elevated norepinephrine and demonstrate exaggerated stress reactions (Wong et al., 2000). Additionally, vulnerability from childhood trauma or adversity may be moderated by polymorphisms in the corticotropin-releasing factor type 1 receptor gene (Bradley et al., 2008). Gene–stress interactions impacting the risk of MDD can be found across neurotransmitter systems (aan het Rot, Mathew, & Charney, 2009) supporting the notion of a complex diathesis–stress model of chronic depression.

There is evidence for an interaction between environment and genes, inasmuch as genetic polymorphisms moderate the likelihood of whether or not an individual develops depression in relation to life stress, including early adversity or trauma (Caspi et al. 2003). It thus appears that interactions between genetic diathesis and environmental influences throughout the lifespan together may underlie depression vulnerability in a good number of chronically depressed patients (Caspi et al., 2003; Heim & Binder, 2012). It is now well accepted that genetic diathesis (genes, sex, personality, family history) and environmental influences (stress, abuse, neglect, chronic psychological insults) across the lifespan together likely underlie vulnerability for depression (Kendler, Gardner, & Prescott, 2002; Merikangas & Swendsen, 1997; Nestler et al., 2002). Heim and colleagues (Heim & Binder, 2012; Heim et al., 2009) in their groundbreaking review of human research regarding the link between early life stress and depression, documented how childhood trauma is associated with persistent sensitization of the stress responses as well as altered dynamics of the hypothalamic-pituitary-adrenal axis, which in turn is related

Interactions between genetic and environmental influences may underlie vulnerability to depression

to symptoms of depression. Based on a massive review of the literature, Heim and Binder (2012) suggest that childhood trauma is associated with sensitization of the neuroendocrine stress response, glucocorticoid resistance, increased central corticotropin-releasing factor activity, immune activation, and reduced hippocampal volume, closely paralleling several of the neuroendocrine features of depression. They propose that neuroendocrine changes secondary to early-life stress increase the risk of developing depression in response to stress, potentially due to failure of a connected neural circuitry implicated in emotional, neuroendocrine, and autonomic control to compensate in response to challenge. Heim et al. (2009) claim there may be subgroups of depression that are biologically distinct, dependent on the presence or absence of childhood trauma (interacting with other risk factors), which are responsive to different types of treatments. They further hypothesize that successful treatments normalize this circuitry. These treatments may be pharmacological or psychotherapeutic in nature.

2.1.7   Glutamate

Although much of the research focus to date has been on the monoaminergic system, accumulating evidence suggests that the **glutamatergic system** also plays an important role in the neurobiology and treatment of depression. For example, there is research demonstrating alterations in glutamate levels of blood and cerebrospinal fluid in patients with MDD. Kim and colleagues (Kim, Schmid-Burgk, Claus, & Kornhuber, 1982) have reported that serum levels of glutamate in patients with depression were significantly higher than those of healthy controls. There is also a positive correlation between plasma glutamate levels and severity of depressive symptoms found in patients with MDD (Mitani et al., 2006). It also seems that determination of blood levels of glutamate may be a biomarker for MDD. Furthermore, a number of drugs that can affect glutamatergic neurotransmission exhibit antidepressant-like activities in animal models of depression. Specifically, the noncompetitive N-methyl D-aspartate (NMDA) receptor antagonist **ketamine** acts on the glutamatergic system and has demonstrated therapeutic drug for treatment-resistant patients with MDD (Hashimoto, 2009). Additional research in this area is required, but the glutamatergic system appears to be a promising model for development.

> Glutamate levels may be positively related to MDD diagnosis

2.1.8   Brain Structure

Brain-imaging technologies, such as magnetic resonance imaging (MRI) and functional MRI (fMRI), have shown that the brains of people who have depression are structurally and functionally different than those of people without depression. For example, patients with recurrent MDD have smaller hippocampi, which may explain reported memory problems in those with depression. Other areas of the brains of depressed patients may be smaller as well, including the anterior cingulate cortex, orbitofrontal cortex, and prefrontal cortex (Hajek, Kozeny, Kopecek, Alda, & Höschl, 2008). Neuroimaging investigations into adult MDD have revealed dysfunction in frontal regions

> Brains of depressed patients appear to be structurally different from nondepressed individuals

including medial, orbital, dorsolateral, and ventrolateral prefrontal cortex as well as the anterior cingulate cortex (Price & Drevets, 2012). These structural changes are hypothesized to augment appraisal of threat and may contribute to relapse. Many of these changes in the brain remain even when the patient is in remission from active depression. One hypothesis is that these structural brain changes may be a part of what contributes to the high relapse rates for people with chronic depressive disorders. The brains of young depressed patients were examined by Vilgis and colleagues (Vilgis, Chin, Silk, Cunnington, & Vance, 2014) who discovered that patients with DD as compared with normal controls, showed less activation in left frontal regions including left ventrolateral and dorsolateral prefrontal cortices during mental rotation. Medial frontal regions including the dorsomedial prefrontal cortex, anterior cingulate cortex, and frontal pole also showed relatively reduced activation. These researchers believe the pathophysiology of depressive disorders extends to DD as a risk factor for MDD and exhibits continuity over the lifespan.

2.2   Psychological Models

Psychology does not have the unified approach to the etiology of depression that is found in biology, but there are psychological models that provide theories for why patients become depressed. Fewer psychological models focus on the development and maintenance of PDD. I will focus here only on psychological models, theories, or approaches that specifically address PDD and upon which empirically supported psychotherapeutic interventions have been developed and disseminated.

The psychological models described below can be considered theoretically integrated approaches to PDD in that they each utilize common factors of multiple theories into a broader framework for understanding and treating PDD. Beckham proposed that

Psychological models of depression often integrate multiple theories

> depression may be viewed as a homeostatic system to the extent that it involves many different components of a patient's life and consists of feedback loops of reciprocal maintaining processes among those components. According to this model the effect of psychotherapy in altering one element of the depressive homeostasis quickly spreads to other elements in the depressive system. (Beckham, 1990, p. 211)

Beckham further speculated that this might help explain why different treatment approaches for depression may be equally effective. Beckham proposes that different treatments may disturb the homeostatic balance of depression by intervening in different areas: cognitive, affective, interpersonal, behavioral, or biological. This way of thinking holds promise in psychology for a comprehensive framework of theoretical integration in our approach to PDD, but we are not there yet. Below are the currently held models of PDD that also have corresponding well-developed and demonstrated treatment approaches.

2.2.1   Interpersonal Models

Interpersonal characteristics and behaviors have been theorized to play an important role in the development and maintenance of PDD, and a number of researchers have characterized depression as a paucity of social skills or interactions (Pettit & Joiner, 2005). According to this model, a depressed patient's negative interpersonal behaviors or lack of interpersonal skills cause others to reject them or avoid them in predictable ways or lead to a lack of rewarding interactions and behaviors with associated negative impact on mood. Interpersonal skill deficits, such as lack of assertiveness, self-centeredness, excessive self-revelation, or avoidance behaviors have been found in depressed patients and are theorized to contribute to depressive symptoms and their maintenance (Hames, Hagan, & Joiner, 2013). In describing the development of PDD specifically, interpersonal theorists posit that in an escalating cycle, depressed individuals, who desperately want positive interactions or reassurance from others, start to make an increasing number of requests for reassurance, and those others to whom those requests are made, start to negatively evaluate, avoid, and reject the depressed individual. Depression symptoms worsen as a result of others' rejection and avoidance and can become perpetuating, eventually leading to PDD (Hames et al., 2013; Markowitz, 2003).

> IPT focuses on interpersonal issues associated with depressive symptoms

Interpersonal Therapy (IPT) approaches are designed to help address and stop this negative spiral, increase interpersonal skills such as appropriate assertiveness, and challenge and change the chronically depressed patient's identity or "role" as a depressed, unhappy, ineffective person. IPT was originally developed by Klerman and colleagues (Klerman, Weissman, Rounsaville, & Chevron, 1984) for use with depressed patients and has been revised for use with patients with DD (Markowitz, 1998, 2003; Pettit & Joiner, 2005). IPT is based on the interpersonal model of depression and was also informed by psychodynamic and social processes. Klerman et al. (1984) identified four social situations of vulnerability for the onset of depression and described how lack of skills in navigating such situations leads to depression. These four primary interpersonal areas are (1) grief – specifically the death of a significant individual; (2) role disputes – conflict with another individual about interpersonal roles; (3) role transitions – conflicts with another individual about change in status, such as divorce or marriage; and (4) interpersonal deficits – such as lack of social skills or paucity of interpersonal relationships. The therapeutic approach of IPT involves helping the patient identify and learn strategies to resolve or overcome each interpersonal difficulty or conflict.

> The "role" or identity of the depressive patient can help maintain depression

2.2.2   Learning and Behavioral Models

> Learning or behavioral models emphasize the role of the environment in depression

Behavioral and learning models of depression emphasize the role of the environment in shaping behavior (Abreu & Santos, 2008; Lewinsohn, 1979). Thus the focus is on observable behavior and the conditions in which individuals learn behavior. Traditional **classical conditioning**, **operant conditioning**, and **social learning theory** paradigms are all used to explain the development and maintenance of depression.

Behavioral and learning theory approaches to depression hypothesize that to understand behavioral variations observed in depressed clients, it is necessary to understand the variables responsible for the cause and maintenance of the depressive feelings of the patient. This process can be reached by identifying the "depressive" contingencies, which involves identifying the antecedent events and consequences of the depressive behaviors of interest. Classical conditioning theories explore the role of paired association of stimuli with negative emotional states. Social learning theory addresses how depression may also be learned via imitation or modeling of depressive behaviors or emotions. Operant conditioning theories hypothesize that removal of positive reinforcers from the environment leads to further social withdrawal and further reductions in positive reinforcement and, ultimately, depression. Additionally, learning theories explore how depression may develop in response to reinforcement by others of depressed behaviors, either intentionally or unintentionally.

Ferster (1973) proposed that depression could be explained by the reduced frequency of positively reinforcing behaviors that serve to control the patient's environment. This occurs, according to Ferster (1973), because characteristics of the depressed person such as excessive crying, irritability, and self-criticism lead to the loss of other types of activities. This idea integrates the interpersonal characteristics and behaviors of the depressed patient with behavioral theory. Ferster proposed that the origin and maintenance of depressive symptoms is due not only to the absence of reinforcers but also to the presence of avoidant behaviors that maintain a very marked pattern of behavioral inhibition. This concept is relatable to PDD patients' lack of assertive interpersonal behaviors as described in IPT and CBASP.

Ferster explained depression as reduced positively reinforcing behaviors and increased avoidant behaviors

Lewinsohn and Talkington (1979) presented a model similar to Ferster's in that it recognized that depressive symptoms could be the result of a reduction of positively reinforced behaviors. Lewinsohn coined the phrase **low rate of response-contingent positive reinforcement** to refer to this characteristic in depressed patients (Lewinsohn & Talkington, 1979). According to Lewinsohn, there are three ways to explain the low rates of response-contingent positive responses of depressed patients. One is that events for the depressed patient are simply no longer positively reinforcing. Another is that the patient's environment has changed so that the reinforcer is not available, and the third situation occurs when the reinforcer is still available in the environment, but the individual no longer has the ability to access it. All three situations would lead to maintenance of depression.

In 2001, Martell and colleagues (Martell, Addis, & Jacobson, 2001) released a handbook on behavior analysis with a treatment of depression called **behavioral activation** (BA) based on behavioral theory. These researchers proposed that depression results from problems in the patient's interaction with the environment that result in the individual "not engaging in behaviors that would be positively reinforced and that would allow that individual to exert control over the environment" (Martell et al., 2001, p. 26). They proposed that learning to approach and cope with aversive situations was important to help depressed patients improve, and that such problem solving would result in positive reinforcement. According to Jacobson, Martell, and Dimidjian (2001), the work of the behavioral therapist was to try to map which contingencies are maintaining the depressive behaviors of the patient and attempt to change

Martell promoted that avoidant behaviors and absence of approach behaviors maintain depression

them. Jacobson highlighted the importance of the contingences of avoidance and escape behaviors, as well as the negative impact of complaining and other unpleasant interpersonal behaviors of depressed patients. The BA therapy approach highlights that in the depressed patient, these behaviors would be negatively reinforced and would inhibit positively reinforced behaviors from being manifested. Therefore, facing the aversive situations would be an important part of overthrowing depression.

Seligman proposed the importance of learned helplessness in the development of depression

The **learned helplessness theory** of depression was developed by Martin Seligman (Seligman, 1973) and describes the etiology of depression as occurring when an individual learns that their attempts to escape negative situations make no difference. This research was originally conducted with dogs but was extended to humans. Seligman proposed that people give up trying to influence their environment because they have learned that they are helpless, as a consequence of having no control over what happens to them. This behavioral explanation can also integrate the fact that humans have negative cognitions that develop in response to such environmental conditions, which leads us to important developments in cognition and depression.

Learned helplessness occurs when one learns that behaviors have no impact on the environment

2.2.3   Cognitive and Integrative Models

Integrative expansions of the models above describe the feedback loops of predisposing factors such as biological vulnerabilities or protections, environmental events, disruption of patterned or learned behaviors, reduction in positive reinforcement or increase in aversive experiences, increased negative self-awareness or self-focus, increased dysphoria, and negative emotional, behavioral, cognitive, interpersonal, and somatic consequences (Lewinsohn, Hoberman, Teri, & Hautzinger, 1985). For instance, behavioral theories have been enriched by the inclusion of cognitive factors as well as interpersonal factors. Abramson and colleagues (Abramson, Seligman, & Teasdale, 1978) introduced a cognitive version of the learned helplessness theory, by reformulating it in terms of how individuals explain the cause of an event – termed their **attributional style**. This style was presumed to have three dimensions: locus (internal or external), stability (stable or transient), and causation (global or specific). In this cognitive version, the development of learned behavior depends on a combination of a negative environmental event and attribution of the negative event to an external, unstable, and specific cause.

Attributional style describes the way an individual explains the cause of an event

Rehm proposed that deficits in self-control or self-management were associated with depression

Rehm's theory of self-control (Rehm, 1977) and Lewinsohn's theory of self-awareness (Lewinsohn, Mischel, Chaplin, & Barton, 1980) are additional examples of the integration of theories. Rehm's self-control theory (Rehm, 1977) integrates elements of the cognitive and behavioral theories proposed by Beck, Lewinsohn, and Seligman. Rehm proposed a self-control model of depression based on the three processes included in a feedback loop model of self-control: self-monitoring, self-evaluation, and self-reinforcement. In this model, depression is characterized as the result of deficits in these processes of self-control. This theory is considered to be a diathesis–stress model and describes depression as a loss of association between external reinforcers and the control of behavior. Lewinsohn's self-awareness theory (Lewinsohn et al., 1980) proposes that there is an increase in depressed patients' self-awareness of their inability to cope, which causes more distress in their lives, thus leading to additional depressive symptoms.

Further development of the cognitive theories of depression is associated with the work of Aaron Beck (Beck, 1991), Albert Ellis (Ellis & Grieger, 1977), and with Jeffrey Young's **schema therapy** (Young, Klosko, & Weishaar, 2003). **Cognitive theories** focus on the role of patients' thoughts, beliefs, and schemas in the development and maintenance of depression. Current cognitive theories regarding PDD are typically integrative and, depending upon the specific intervention, can incorporate behavioral, interpersonal, psychodynamic, and attachment components, as in schema therapy. Cognitive-based theories all maintain that depression results from systematic negative bias in thinking processes and that these changes in thinking precede the onset of depressed mood and facilitate maintenance of depression. Emotional, behavioral, and potentially even physical symptoms are seen as a result of errors or abnormalities in thinking that are different from those of nondepressed individuals.

Beck (1987) proposed that depressed individuals appraise events in a negative manner, and this distorted view or interpretation of events leads to distorted emotional conditions such as depression. He identified three mechanisms responsible for depression: (1) the **cognitive triad** of negative automatic thinking, (2) **negative self-schemas**, and (3) **errors in logical thinking** or information processing. The negative cognitive triad refers to the tendency for depressed patients to have a negative view of themselves, the world, and the future. These negative thoughts are well rehearsed and spontaneous; they are automatic for the patient and are rarely examined or questioned. According to Beck (1987), depressed patients tend to view themselves as worthless, inadequate, and helpless, and then also interpret the world as negative and unhelpful, and the future as hopeless. As these components interact, they are hypothesized to interfere with normal cognitive processing and lead to impairments in memory and problem solving, thus perpetuating the difficulties. Beck also described a negative self-schema as an important component of depression and believed that depressed patients possess a set of beliefs about themselves that are essentially negative and pessimistic. These negative schemas could be acquired in childhood as a result of trauma or neglect or other negative experiences. These events alone, however, may not be enough to lead to depression. Stressful life events are also required to "activate" these negative schemas from earlier in life. This is yet another example of the diathesis–stress model of depression. Once the negative schema is activated, the hypothesis is that the previous negative and illogical thoughts or cognitive biases will begin to dominant thinking, ultimately leading to depression. These are the errors in logical thinking that Beck described as the final mechanism for depressed mood. Beck proposed that patients with activated negative self-schemas become prone to making logical errors in thinking or information processing. Such patients focus selectively on certain aspects of a situation or the environment, while systematically ignoring other features, and this results in erroneous information processing.

Schema therapy originally developed as an expansion of traditional cognitive behavioral theory and therapy. The theoretical model of schema therapy assumes that patients with psychological problems such as depression are

Cognitive model focuses on role of thoughts, schemas, and beliefs in development and maintenance of depression

The negative self-schema of depressed patients is a set of negative and pessimistic self-beliefs characterized by a distinct set of **early maladaptive schemas** (EMSs; Young et al., 2003). These schemas determine the way patients perceive the world, themselves, and others, and can have a powerful impact on emotions, behaviors, and sensations. According to Young, changing the schemas of depressed patients can change symptoms, and the reduction in depressive symptoms can then positively impact schemas, and/or schemas can simultaneously change with depressive symptoms, which is the mechanism that has been most clearly supported by study reports in the literature (Renner et al., 2018).

Renner developed a cognitive schema model of chronic depression

Renner and colleagues (Renner, Arntz, Leeuw, & Huibers, 2013) developed a cognitive schema model of chronic depression that describes the interplay between four identified risk factors for chronic depression. These four risk factors have received the most consistent support from study reports in the literature and include early adversity, personality pathology, cognitive factors, and interpersonal factors. In Renner's integrative model, EMSs and dysfunctional thoughts and attitudes mediate the effect of early adversity on depression. These schemas are triggered by current environmental events such as loss or failure and are maintained by avoidance-related coping strategies and interpersonal behaviors that reinforce the schemas. Such interpersonal avoidance behaviors, such as lack of assertiveness, then lead to lack of positive social interactions and reinforcement and maintenance of depression.

McCullough (McCullough, 2000; McCullough, Schramm, & Penberthy, 2015) developed a model of chronic depression that integrates developmental, learning, cognitive, interpersonal theory, and behavioral analysis. CBASP presents an etiological premise that PDD arises, in part, as a result of a developmental history characterized by significant interpersonal trauma (e.g., physical and/or sexual abuse) or a low-grade, continuous stream of psychological insults (e.g., punishment or rejection of some form). The trauma and insults, through the process of classical conditioning, lead to feelings of not being emotionally safe and not trusting others – a lack of felt emotional safety on the part of the depressed patient. Operant conditioning then results in social withdrawal and avoidance behaviors of the depressed patient, which perpetuates the paucity of social interactions or interpersonally rewarding interactions. This leads to cognitive-emotional developmental arrest within the depressed patient, with negative impacts on social, cognitive, and emotional functioning, and ultimately to what McCullough (2000), borrowing a developmental term from Piaget, calls **preoperational functioning**. The adult patient

CBASP conceptualizes PDD as an interpersonal learning derailment

is hypothesized to function at a cognitive-emotional level resembling that of a preoperational child. This developmental derailment is characterized by a lack of causal awareness and pervasive egocentrism in the depressive patient that often results in a presentation of poor functioning and low motivation for change. McCullough (2000) proposed that a lack of awareness of interpersonal impact, inability to generate genuine empathy, and poor interpersonal problem-solving skills were associated with persistent depression. Patients with PDD are conceptualized as having rigidly intrapersonally closed systems, with the current environment and individuals in it no longer informing them. Avoidance behavior combined with the derailment described above is hypothesized to lead to helplessness, hopelessness, and maintenance of depressed mood (McCullough et al., 2015).

The CBASP model takes a person-by-environment perspective in modifying depressive symptoms based on the theorized etiology described above (McCullough, 2000, 2012b). This means that the environment and the person interact to create the disorder and must both be addressed to treat the disorder. The CBASP model proposes that PDD patients often perceive that causal influences in their lives are beyond their control. Research in this area supports the suggestion that PDD patients feel unsafe, avoid others, demonstrate maladaptive interpersonal styles, have poor abilities to use a problem-focused coping style, and are often perceptually disconnected from feedback in their interpersonal environment (Locke et al., 2017; Negt et al., 2016). Increasing the depressed patient's feelings of emotional safety and increasing their awareness and abilities regarding their interpersonal impact on others and the environment – what McCullough terms **perceived functionality** – are the two primary goals of CBASP. The CBASP model proposes that the interpersonal fear driving patient avoidance, the central theme in many interpersonal failures, must be counter-conditioned. This is done by aiding the patient in discriminating their experiences with a helpful, caring psychotherapist, from those experiences with harmful significant others, to create a sense of felt interpersonal safety and effective appropriate approach behavior that can then be generalized outside of the therapy setting.

Addressing lack of felt emotional safety and poor interpersonal functioning are part of the CBASP

The second major component of CBASP focuses on an interpersonal problem-solving tool called **situational analysis** (SA), which is used in session to help a patient actively re-experience an interpersonal encounter (McCullough, 2000). The goal is to elicit the original cognitions and emotions during the target situation. This involves teaching the depressed patient to mindfully isolate a moment in time, describe it in exclusively behavioral terms, and identify the interpersonal situational outcome. The goal of this exercise is to help depressed patients identify alternative ways of behaving and thinking that would lead to more desirable consequences, while also simultaneously beginning to recognize their own roles in their dilemma. Recognizing their stimulus value in the interpersonal context and becoming more interpersonally mindful is hypothesized to allow the person with chronic depression to amend how they interact with stressful interpersonal situations. New ways of behaving interpersonally are hypothesized to lead to desirable outcomes, reinforce effective problem-solving skills, and allow the patient to perceive their contingent relationship with the environment (McCullough, 2000, 2006, 2012b). Through these means, the depressed patient is hypothesized to acquire the ability to recognize and begin to change the interpersonal consequences of their behavior.

2.2.4   Mindfulness-Based Models

Researchers have proposed that previously depressed individuals are more vulnerable to relapse in the face of a small negative change in mood (Mickalak, Holz, & Teismann, 2011). The hypothesis is that previously depressed individuals may have an increased tendency for a ruminative response style, which makes them more vulnerable to becoming depressed again when faced with even a small change in mood. Mindfulness-based models combine components of **cognitive behavior therapy** (CBT) and traditional mindfulness

Some researchers propose that depression relapse is caused in part by a ruminative response style

Mindfulness is described as paying attention in a particular way, in present moment and without judgment

theory with the hypothesis that teaching patients how to me mindful – that is, to intentionally pay attention in the present moment without judgment – will help reduce ruminative thinking and thus prevent depressive relapse. **Mindfulness-based cognitive therapy** (MBCT; Segal, Williams, & Teasdale, 2013), which grew out of CBT and mindfulness theory, has been shown to help patients quiet their repetitive upsetting thoughts or ruminations and detach from depression-related thoughts and feelings. MBCT theorizes that teaching previously depressed patients mindfulness skills allows them to be more aware of their thoughts, feelings, and sensations, and to change the way they relate to them, thus preventing relapse (MacKenzie & Kocovski, 2016).

Diagnosis and Treatment Indications

PDD is conceptualized differently from acute or episodic depression, and effective psychotherapeutic approaches to PDD differ from the approaches for those. Compared with an acute or episodic course, PDD is associated with earlier onset, increased rates of abuse and adverse early experiences (Klein & Santiago, 2003); increased comorbidities, especially personality disorders (Angst et al., 2009); and poor social and interpersonal adjustment (Ley et al., 2011). PDD patients may need more intense and longer courses of treatment (Cuijpers, van Straten, et al., 2010) or treatments designed specifically for their needs (McCullough, 2000, 2006). Medical disorders must also be evaluated, since some medical conditions can present with depressive symptoms and may respond to treatment of the underlying medical condition (Goodwin, 2006). The age of onset, severity of depressive symptoms, developmental trauma history, current interpersonal functioning, and dysfunctional schemas and cognitions should be evaluated and considered when making treatment recommendations, since these factors may be used to direct a more effective treatment. A flowchart of this approach to diagnosis and treatment can be found in Figure 2. Additional information related to aspects of the flowchart is presented in the next paragraphs.

> **Differentiating PDD from acute or episodic depression is important for determining treatment approach**

The initial assessment should be based on a detailed history, including diagnostic interview and physical examination if possible, with thorough blood work checking for medical issues that may be contributing to the depressive symptoms. Depression is a clinical diagnosis, based on the patient's history and physical findings. No diagnostic laboratory tests are available to diagnose PDD, but focused laboratory studies may be useful to identify and treat medical illnesses or side effects from medications that may present as depression, be associated with depression, or worsen depression.

3.1   Motivation or Readiness to Change

It is important to determine the patient's **motivation to change** or readiness to engage in treatment. Readiness to change can be assessed directly or inferred based on patient behaviors and statements. Treatment history should include the types of any antidepressants used, dose, compliance, response to treatment, and side effects experienced. Treatment history should also include the type of psychotherapy or supportive services obtained, if any, and the degree of engagement, belief in efficacy, and treatment response. Reasons for discontinuing prior psychotherapy should also be assessed, and it is important to

> **Patient motivation, treatment history, and engagement should be used to inform the approach used**

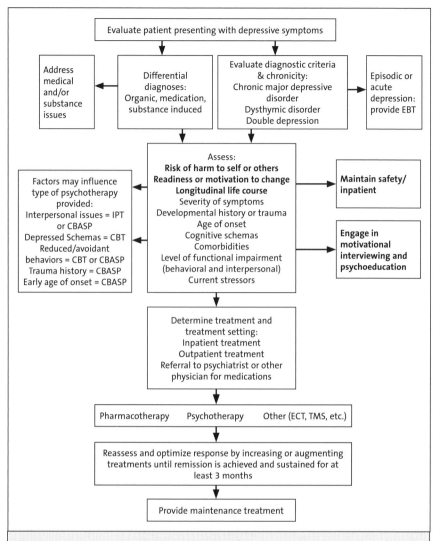

Figure 2
Diagnosis and treatment algorithm for persistent depressive disorder (PDD).
CBASP = cognitive behavioral analysis system of psychotherapy; CBT = cognitive
behavior therapy; EBT = evidence based therapy; ECT = electroconvulsive
therapy; IPT = interpersonal psychotherapy; TMS = transcranial magnetic
stimulation.

proactively monitor and assess any recurrence of these problems. Compliance issues can interfere with effective implementation of treatment and may need to be addressed via additional interventions, such as motivational interviewing to clarify ambivalence and advance readiness to change and increase adherence to treatments, or through psychoeducational interventions to help provide information and support (Donker, Griffiths, Cuijpers, & Christensen, 2009). The CBASP approach includes proactive techniques to address therapy-interfering behaviors of the patient and help increase engagement of the patient (McCullough, 2006).

3.2   Longitudinal Life Course

Evaluation of the patient's history should take into consideration age of onset of depression, the relationship of depressive symptoms to significant life events, change in season (seasonal affective disorder), peripartum period, and phase of menstrual cycle. Developmental history including past or current trauma or stress, symptom dimensions, symptom severity, comorbid psychiatric and medical conditions (particularly comorbid substance abuse), the risk of harm to self or others, level of functioning, and the socio-cultural-spiritual milieu of the patient should also be assessed. Assessment of strengths and resources is important to understand positive factors that may be drawn upon in treatment. This information can inform and guide the therapeutic approach and inform the nature of the therapeutic relationship and the expectations of the patient (Keller et al., 2000; McCullough et al., 2016a). Specifically, if the patient has failed repeated treatment approaches, the therapist should be aware of possible learned helplessness and the possible subsequent negative impact upon the patient's motivation to engage in therapy.

The patient's illness and treatment course, including remissions and recurrences, may inform treatment

3.3   Symptom Severity and Suicide Risk

Ideally, once the diagnosis of PDD is determined, the severity of symptoms can be assessed via a standardized scale, which is then used throughout treatment to evaluate progress. The construct of severity can be in relation to patient risk for suicidal and homicidal behavior (Sokero et al., 2005) and/or operationally defined and conceptualized in terms of mild, moderate, and severe depressive symptoms (Goethe, Fischer, & Wright, 1993). The presence of suicidal ideation, psychotic symptoms, severe anxiety, panic attacks, and alcohol or substance abuse, all of which increases the risk of suicide, should be evaluated. A suicidal risk inventory or other assessment such as the BHS (Beck, Weissman, Lester, & Trexler, 1974), which has demonstrated correlations with suicide risk, is recommended to evaluate suicidal risk (Wolfe et al., 2017). Evaluation should include history of past suicide attempts including the nature of those attempts and any history of suicide in the patient's family history. It is also important to inquire about the degree to which the patient intends to act on any suicidal ideation and the extent to which the patient has made plans or begun to prepare for suicide, and their access to means and opportunity. Patients who express suicidal or homicidal ideation, intention, or plans require close monitoring. Suicidal patients must be provided with safety first, and this may mean providing inpatient treatment along with medications and safety precautions before psychotherapy begins. Patients with catatonic depression or who are demonstrating paranoid or psychotic symptoms may also need to be triaged for hospitalization, medication management, or other biological intervention prior to being able to meaningfully participate in effective psychotherapy.

Severity of depressive symptoms is an important consideration in treatment planning for PDD

Suicide risk must be assessed and monitored for patients with PDD: with suicide risk inventory or the BHS

Patients who are acutely catatonic, paranoid, or delusional may not be appropriate for psychotherapy for PDD

Data are mixed regarding the most effective treatments for various levels of severity of depression (i.e., mild, moderate, severe). It has been asserted that psychotherapy or medication may be equally effective for patients with mild or moderate depression, but that for patients with severe depression, medication is more effective (Fournier et al., 2010). However, in an analysis of four studies examining the use of medication or CBT for severely depressed patients, researchers found a small, but not statistically significant advantage of CBT alone over medication alone (DeRubeis, Gelfand, Tang, & Simons, 1999). Another study (Keller et al., 2000) compared CBASP with medication in a PDD population and demonstrated that both worked equally well and, when combined, their effect was additive. In this study medication had a greater impact during the first 4 weeks, and psychotherapy had more of an impact during the last 8 weeks of treatment. The UK's National Institute for Health and Care Excellence (NICE) clinical guidelines of the British Psychological Society (National Collaborating Centre for Mental Health, 2010) recommend that clinicians provide a combination of antidepressant and a high-intensity psychological intervention for people with moderate or severe depression. Because chronic depression also tends to be more severe (Torpey & Klein, 2008), I recommend that patients diagnosed with PDD of any severity level receive treatment with both pharmacotherapy and psychotherapy.

> **Severity of depression is an important concept to evaluate in PDD patients**

3.4   Onset Age

Compared with patients with late-onset PDD, those with early-onset PDD tend to have longer episodes of major depression, greater likelihood of family history of mood disorder, and higher rates of personality disorders, lifetime substance abuse, and childhood adversity (Garyfallos et al., 1999). They use fewer problem-solving coping skills and are less resilient overall (McCullough et al., 1990). Schramm et al. (2011) found that PDD outpatients with early-onset depression responded significantly better to CBASP than IPT, mean BDI score = 10.79 for CBASP, vs. 21.27 for IPT; $F(1,26) = 4.34$, $p = .047$, ES_{IPT-CM}: $d = .87$. There was a statistically significant difference between CBASP and IPT regarding response rates at posttreatment: 64.3% vs. 26.7%, $\chi^2(1) = 4.144$, $p = .042$, favoring therapy with CBASP. Remission rates also differed significantly between the two groups, with higher rates for the CBASP patients versus those receiving IPT: Intent-to-treat sample: CBASP: 57.1% vs. IPT: 20.0%, $\chi^2(1) = 4.24$, $p = .039$. Based on these limited results, CBASP appears to be a preferred approach for patients presenting early-onset PDD, and thus assessing for onset age is important.

> **CBASP may be more effective than IPT for early-onset depression**

There are mixed findings regarding response to antidepressant medications and age of onset in PDD. Patients with longer episodes of depression have lower remission rates in response to citalopram and may require multiple trials of medications before achieving remission (Warden et al., 2007). In the STAR*D study, remission with medication alone was less likely for patients with a longer time since first episode onset, a longer length of current MDE, or more medical and psychiatric comorbidities (Warden et al., 2007).

3.5   Trauma History

Trauma during childhood or later in life has been hypothesized to play a role in the development of PDD (Caspi et al., 2003; Heim & Binder, 2012). Retrospective and prospective studies have found increased rates of traumatic events, especially childhood trauma, in patients with PDD (Klein, Roniger, Schweiger, Späth, & Brodbeck, 2015). Personality disorders also have been associated with childhood trauma (Tyrka, Wyche, Kelly, Price, & Carpenter, 2009). It is no surprise then that PDD is often comorbid with personality disorders. Compared with patients with episodic depression, patients with PDD are twice as likely to have comorbid personality disorders (Rothschild & Zimmerman, 2002). Researchers have hypothesized that since the comorbidity of depression with personality disorders is much higher than expected by chance alone; the high rates may be due to the common underlying factor of childhood trauma (Kounou et al., 2013).

There are increased rates of both childhood trauma and personality disorders in PDD

Early trauma may negatively impact individuals by arresting normal biological, interpersonal, and psychological development. PDD patients frequently describe a developmental history rife with instances of either repeated psychological insults or serious psychological or physical trauma (McCullough et al., 2015). These early experiences may lead to learned fear, interpersonal avoidance, and retreat with disastrous interpersonal-social consequences. McCullough et al. (2015) propose that an additional consequence of early trauma may be a concomitant derailment of normal cognitive-emotional maturational growth, in the form of arrested cognitive-emotional development. PDD patients may be unaware that their thought and behavior patterns keep them perceptually disconnected from the environment. This means that they may be less responsive to environmental consequences and feedback.

Preoperational thinking may characterize the PDD patient, especially those with histories of early trauma

The lack of cognitive capacity in the interpersonal-social arena of PDD due to early traumas may explain why it has traditionally been so challenging to treat these patients. Historically, outcome research has demonstrated that chronic depression is a difficult condition to treat with CBT, especially when it is characterized by early onset or early trauma (Moore & Garland, 2003). Cuijpers, Smit, Bohlmeijer, Hollon, and Andersson (2010) conducted a meta-analysis of psychotherapy for MDD and DD and concluded that psychotherapy is effective in the treatment of PDD and DD but probably less so than pharmacotherapy. However, most of the studies reviewed had methodological weaknesses such as very short courses of psychotherapy.

Riso and Newman (2003) describe the impact of early trauma as increasing the likelihood of entrenched negative core beliefs or EMSs, which tend to be rigid and overgeneralized. In fact, the concept of EMS in CBT was developed to help patients with severe interpersonal problems and personality disorders. Patients with EMSs are more likely to have difficulty establishing a productive therapeutic alliance and face greater challenges in using the CBT or schema therapy model. In fact, the goal of schema therapy is to decrease the impact of these dysfunctional schemas and replace them with functional ones (Renner et al., 2018). Schema therapy for PDD has grown out of the need to address early trauma but has very limited research evidence to date.

Early trauma may lead to increased EMSs in PDD

CBASP was designed with the interpersonal-social limitations of the PDD patient in mind and has demonstrated techniques to address these develop-

CBASP for PDD patients with early trauma has been shown to be effective

mental limitations (McCullough, 2000). In a large reanalysis study, Nemeroff et al. (2003) demonstrated that for a group of 681 chronically depressed patients with early childhood trauma, CBASP was particularly effective. Completer analysis using logistic modeling revealed a significantly higher remission rate in the patients with chronic forms of major depression and early life trauma treated with CBASP compared with those receiving nefazodone (Wald χ^2 = 6.8912, df = 1, p = .0087). The superiority of CBASP (with or without nefazodone) for patients reporting early life trauma persisted when the analyses were controlled for sex, age, race, and depression severity at baseline (Nemeroff et al., 2003).

A history of adverse childhood experiences has been associated with decreased responsiveness to pharmacological treatment in patients with DD and MDD (Williams, Debattista, Duchemin, Schatzberg, & Nemeroff, 2016).

3.6 Co-Occurring Disorders or Medical Comorbidities

PDD often co-occurs with other disorders

PDD may often occur with other psychiatric disorders, and it is important to take into consideration these comorbidities when planning treatment. A full discussion of all possible comorbidities that may occur with PDD is beyond the scope of this book, but some of the more common ones include other depressive disorders (Klein et al., 2008), personality disorders, anxiety including posttraumatic stress disorder, GAD, obsessive-compulsive disorder, and substance abuse disorders (Thaipisuttikul, Ittasaku, Waleeprakhon, Wisajun, & Jullagate, 2014) as well as an assortment of medical conditions, such as chronic fatigue syndrome, fibromyalgia, headaches, and irritable bowel syndrome (Kang et al., 2015). It is also important to rule out or identify medical conditions that may be causing or contributing to symptoms of depression, such as thyroid disease or sleep disorders (Gelenberg, Kocsis, McCullough, Ninan, & Thase, 2006). Researchers have found an elevated bidirectional risk between MDD and chronic medical illnesses (Katon, 2011), which may in part be reflective of common underlying pathophysiological processes involving the proliferation of stress-related psychoneuroimmunological abnormalities (Epstein, Szpindel, & Katzman, 2014).

Ruling out bipolar disorder is an important aspect of the evaluation for PDD. Many patients with bipolar disorder present to clinicians during the depressive phase of the illness and may not report previous hypomanic or manic episodes spontaneously. Obtaining a thorough history from the patient and other sources, such as family members, can provide important clues for diagnosing bipolar disorder. For this reason, it is a good idea to use standardized assessments. Treating bipolar depression as a unipolar disorder can increase the risk that antidepressants may induce manic or hypomanic symptoms (Viktorin et al., 2014). The presence of psychotic features, marked psychomotor retardation, reverse neurovegetative symptoms (excessive sleep and appetite), irritability, anger, family history of bipolar disorder, and early age of onset are clues that the diagnosis of bipolar should be further investigated.

Another reason to assess for comorbidities is that patients with PDD and other psychiatric illness are twice as likely to make suicide attempts than patients without comorbid depression (Dolnak, 2006). It is important to establish which symptoms are overlapping with the depressive diagnosis and which are distinct. If most symptoms are overlapping, then treatment for those symptoms may help improve both disorders (National Collaborating Centre for Mental Health, 2010). If the symptoms are fully distinct, concurrent or sequential treatment that addresses both disorders may be necessary to positively impact the two separate disorders. It is preferable to treat PDD and comorbid disorders concomitantly if possible, as this has been demonstrated to be more effective in promoting improvement in both disorders (Dolnak, 2006).

Comorbidities can increase risk for suicide in depressed patients

4

Treatment

IPT, CBT, and CBASP are three psychotherapies that have been studied in PDD and found to be effective

In the following sections, three empirically supported psychotherapy methods for treating PDD will be presented. I find these to have the most robust research support and have found them to be effective in my work with PDD patients. I have chosen these three systems of therapy because they have been manualized and are supported by a body of empirical data. I will cover IPT for dysthymia and CBT for chronic and persistent depression briefly, and will provide a more detailed exploration of CBASP, keeping in mind that the most effective treatment for PDD appears to be a combination of an empirically supported pharmacotherapy and psychotherapy (Thase et al., 1997). I was trained by Dr. Jim McCullough Jr. and find CBASP to be a very compelling, integrated treatment approach that incorporates components of learning, developmental, interpersonal, and cognitive theory with aspects of interpersonal mindfulness. I find CBASP to be accessible to patients and, most importantly, effective in treating PDD. I continue to use IPT and CBT techniques in my practice, but often find myself using techniques from them in conjunction with CBASP, with CBASP as my primary intervention. While my preference is for CBASP, I realize that other approaches will be more appropriate for some clinicians. My overall goal is that the reader be able to identify and effectively use a psychotherapy approach for PDD patients that works!

Specific versions of IPT (Markowitz, 2003), CBT (Moore & Garland, 2003) and CBASP (McCullough, 2000; McCullough et al., 2015) have been shown to be effective for the treatment of patients with DD and/or chronic MDD. Schema therapy (conceptualized as a form of CBT that concentrates immediately and specifically on schemas and related developmental issues) has demonstrated promise with some initial positive responses (Carter et al., 2013). MBCT has been explored for use in preventing relapse in depression but has less empirical support for treating PDD (Michalak et al., 2015; Segal, Williams, & Teasdale, 2013). Additional psychotherapies may or may not be of benefit, but they do not have research support specifically demonstrating their efficacy in treating patients with PDD.

PDD may require more intense treatment than acute depression

Patients with PDD may respond to psychotherapy, pharmacotherapy, or a combination of both, but treatment response often requires more time, more psychotherapy sessions, and/or higher doses of antidepressant medication than in patients with acute or episodic forms of depression (Keller et al., 2000; Thase et al., 1997). Some patients will respond to pharmacotherapy alone, but many others will benefit from adjunctive psychotherapy (Cuijpers et al., 2012). Unfortunately, we are not yet able to fully personalize treatment.

There are additional somatic treatments typically reserved for what is termed **treatment-resistant depression**, which may overlap with the PDD category (Sackeim, 2001). These treatments include, but are not limited to, ECT, TMS, deep brain stimulation (DBS), and vagal nerve stimulation (VNS). ECT and TMS are the two of these more somatic therapies that have the most research support and have demonstrated usefulness when added to other treatment approaches. These results will be discussed briefly in Section 4.2: Variations and Combinations of Methods (Epstein, Szpindel, & Katzman, 2014).

4.1 Methods of Treatment

4.1.1 Interpersonal Psychotherapy

IPT focuses on interpersonal dysfunction, which, as we have seen, is a significant issue in patients with PDD (see Section 2.2.3: Cognitive and Integrative Models), and thus it is an intuitive treatment fit for this population. IPT was originally designed to treat acute, discrete episodes of depression, and the traditional structure reflects this assumption (Klerman et al., 1984). IPT assumes that depression is a medical illness, is treatable, and not the fault of the patient suffering from depression. In IPT, interpersonal problems are considered to be an additional factor that contributes to the genesis and maintenance of depression (Markowitz, 2003). These interpersonal problems are concerned with either the death of a significant other, an interpersonal role dispute, interpersonal role transition, or interpersonal deficits. The traditional IPT approach assumes that recent life events trigger an acute depressive episode in a vulnerable patient or that the onset of a depressive episode has generated interpersonal difficulties. This is obviously problematic when the depressive disorder has been chronically present, and the traumatic triggering event may have been decades ago, as is often the case in the PDD patient.

IPT focuses on interpersonal dysfunction in the PDD patient

IPT has been adapted for use with chronic depression (IPT-D) by Markowitz (1998, 2003), and that involves helping the patient focus on a role transition from chronic illness to nascent health. Markowitz (1998, 2003) and other IPT researchers propose that many persistently depressed patients feel inferior or fraudulent, as if there were something defective about them or their personality. According to IPT researchers, this chronic feeling of inadequacy is part of what makes intimacy or relationships difficult for these patients. In fact, many patients with PDD present with a paucity of relationships and interpersonal interactions (Locke et al., 2017). Thus, treatment with IPT focuses on helping the patient conceptualize therapy as a role transition from illness to a healthy way of living. Role transition often requires mourning the old, persistently depressed role that the patient is losing, and coming to terms with and gaining mastery over a new healthy role, including learning new interpersonal skills. IPT is typically carried out for an agreed-upon period of time, such as 16 weekly sessions, with a clear endpoint of treatment identified at the outset. Often maintenance visits are scheduled at less frequent intervals after the conclusion of the acute treatment sessions. Treatment is divided into distinct phases: initial, middle, and termination; or assessment, initial sessions,

IPT has been adapted for dysthymic disorder

middle sessions, termination sessions and conclusion of acute treatment, and maintenance sessions (Markowitz, 1998, 2003).

The goals of the IPT therapist are to facilitate independent functioning of the patient, enhance the patent's sense of competence, help the patient get their attachment needs met outside of therapy, and prevent relapse. These goals can be achieved by using strategies such as providing support and positive feedback about the improved functioning and emotional state of the patient and reflecting back the patient's progress and strengths over the course of therapy. Maintenance therapy is recommended because it helps provide a known source of support for the patient (Markowitz & Weissman, 2004). Strategies used during this phase of treatment include anticipating future issues and addressing them proactively, reminding patients of skills and strategies and the fact that they are not alone, and continuing to help patients monitor and proactively address signs of relapse.

Maintenance IPT is recommended to prevent relapse

Ultimately, according to IPT theory (Markowitz, 1998, 2003), success experiences in interpersonal interactions lead to the development of new coping skills and improved mood and sense of competence. Patients may need time and help in adjusting to feeling and functioning better in the world, and IPT researchers thus recommend at least 6 months of continuation of treatment after acute treatment (Markowitz & Weissman, 2004).

IPT Mechanisms of Action

Although IPT has demonstrated efficacy for PDD and related disorders, little is known about its mechanism of action. IPT utilizes a diathesis–stress model of psychiatric illness and integrates two interpersonal frameworks: (1) relational theory, which provides the basis for connecting relationships with mental health; and (2) research on stress, social support, and illness, which informs IPT's specific focus on current interpersonal problems. IPT thus frames therapy around a central interpersonal problem in the patient's life, such as a current crisis or relational predicament that is disrupting social support and increasing interpersonal stress. By mobilizing and working collaboratively with the patient to address this interpersonal problem, IPT seeks to activate several interpersonal change mechanisms in the depressed patient (Markowitz, 1998). These mechanisms include: (1) enhancing social support, (2) decreasing interpersonal stress, (3) facilitating emotional processing, and (4) improving interpersonal skills. In PDD, the focus is typically on the transition of the persistently depressed patient from their role as a depressed patient to being a healthy individual.

IPT helps change the interpersonal problem of the patient or their relationship to that problem or both

IPT researchers theorize that IPT helps the patient resolve the interpersonal problem by altering the problem itself, changing their relationship to the problem, or both (Klerman, Weissman, Rounsaville, & Chevron, 1984). This framework fundamentally distinguishes IPT from many other therapy models, which identify the problem within the patient and seek to change some problematic aspect of the patient's personality, attachment style, or schemas. Thus, IPT researchers should be able to evaluate these mechanistic components and explore the impact on depressive symptoms. The Interpersonal Psychotherapy Outcome Scale (IPOS; Markowitz, Leon, Miller, & Villalobos, 2000) assesses the degree to which patients feel they have solved the focal interpersonal problem in IPT. Using the IPOS, Markowitz and colleagues (Markowitz, Bleiberg,

Christos, & Levitan, 2006) found that symptomatic improvement correlated with DD patients' ratings of degree of resolution of the interpersonal problem. This is a beginning of promising research to explore the mechanisms of IPT and potential impact of interpersonal changes. However, surprisingly little additional research has tested which specific factors mediate change in IPT.

IPT Efficacy and Prognosis

IPT for acute depression has been evaluated in several large randomized controlled trials (RCTs) comparing it with other psychotherapies and pharmacotherapy. There are fewer IPT studies explicitly conducted with PDD patients. In a large meta-analysis of IPT for depression in adults and adolescents, Cuijpers et al. (2011) examined 38 studies including 4,356 patients who reported diagnosable depression. The patient diagnosis identified in 22 studies was MDD, and 3 studies explicitly studied patients with DD. The remaining studies included patients with subthreshold depression. IPT was compared with standard or no treatment in 16 studies, compared with other psychotherapies (CBT, supportive therapy, coping therapy) in 13 studies, and with pharmacotherapy in 10 studies. The overall effect size of the 16 studies that compared IPT and a control group was $d = 0.63$ for IPT, 95% CI, 0.36–0.90. Ten studies of MDD or DD diagnosed patients compared IPT with all other psychotherapies and showed a nonsignificant differential effect size of $d = 0.04$, 95% CI, –0.14 to 0.21, favoring IPT. IPT was compared with CBT and found to have no statistically significant advantage. CBASP was not included in this meta-analysis. Pharmacotherapy was shown to be more effective than IPT ($d = 0.19$, 95% CI, −0.38 to −0.01), and combination treatment was not more effective than IPT alone, although the authors report that the paucity of studies in this category precluded drawing definite conclusions. Combination maintenance treatment with pharmacotherapy and IPT was found to be more effective in preventing relapse than pharmacotherapy alone, odds ratio (OR) = 0.37; 95% CI, 0.19–0.73.

IPT and CBT were not significantly different in their treatment effects

Schramm et al. (2011) conducted an outpatient study to compare 22 sessions of IPT with the same number of sessions of CBASP. In the ITT sample, there was a statistically significant difference between CBASP and IPT with significant improvements posttreatment in the CBASP group versus IPT: 64.3% versus 26.7%, $\chi^2(1) = 4.144$, $p = .042$. Analysis of covariance did not show a significant benefit of CBASP over IPT on the HDRS-24: meant HDRS score of 11.21 in CBASP versus 18.87 in IPT; $F(1,26) = 3.46$, , $p = .074$, ES_{IPT-CM}: $d = .68$; whereas a significantly higher reduction in self-rated depressive symptoms was found in the CBASP group posttreatment versus the IPT group: mean BDI score of 10.79 in CBASP versus 21.27 in IPT; $F(1,26) = 4.34$, $p = .047$, ES_{IPT-CM}: $d = .87$. The remission rates also differed significantly between both groups, with higher rates for the CBASP patients: ITT sample: CBASP: 57.1% versus IPT: 20.0%, $\chi^2(1) = 4.24$, $p = .039$.

Research suggests IPT is less efficacious than pharmacotherapy

The bulk of the research literature to date suggests that IPT is less efficacious than pharmacotherapy and perhaps CBASP, but that IPT has validated effectiveness for treating depression, including PDD (Cuijpers et al., 2011).

It is unclear if maintenance IPT will prevent relapse. Reynolds et al. (1999) examined the efficacy of maintenance nortriptyline hydrochloride and IPT in preventing recurrence of MDE and found recurrence rates over 3 years as follows: nortriptyline and IPT, 20% (95% CI, 4%–36%); nortriptyline and medication clinic visits, 43% (95% CI, 25%–61%); IPT and placebo, 64% (95% CI, 45%–83%); and placebo and medication clinic visits, 90% (95% CI, 79%–100%). Combined treatment with nortriptyline and IPT was superior to IPT and placebo, and showed a trend to superior efficacy over nortriptyline monotherapy (Wald $\chi^2 = 3.56$; $p = .06$). However, Reynolds et al. (2006) found that maintenance IPT is not as effective for patients presenting with only one MDE. In their 2006 study, recurrence rates were 35% among patients receiving paroxetine plus IPT, 37% among those receiving paroxetine plus clinical management sessions, 68% among those receiving placebo plus IPT, and 58% among those receiving placebo plus clinical management sessions. Major depression recurrence rates were lower in the two paroxetine groups than in the placebo groups: relative risk = 0.42, 95% CI, 0.24–0.71; number needed to treat (NNT) = 4, 95% CI, 3–11, respectively. Overall, IPT did not appear to reduce the risk for recurrence.

Maintenance IPT does not appear to reduce risk for recurrence or relapse of depression

4.1.2   Cognitive Behavior Therapy

CBT is one of the most studied and best validated psychotherapy approaches and initially gained prominence as an intervention for acute or episodic depression (Beck, Rush, Shaw, & Emery, 1979). CBT is well evaluated in the treatment of acute depression but significantly less so in the treatment of PDD (Sudak, 2012).

The CBT approach to treatment emphasizes case conceptualization combining information about the patient with what is known about PDD generally (Persons & Bertagnolli, 1999). Although CBT for PDD is not qualitatively different from CBT for acute depression, it does require a different emphasis in the conceptualization as well as greater perseverance on behalf of the patient and therapist (Moore & Garland, 2003). According to Moore and Garland (2003), CBT with PDD patients requires a greater emphasis on addressing hopelessness, helplessness, and perfectionism, early life traumas or adverse events, and modifying EMSs – and, specifically, depressive schemas. A depressive schema is a well-organized and interconnected negative internal representation of self. This schema is believed to develop through early life experiences and to remain dormant or less activated until triggered by negative life events (Beck et al., 1979). Once activated, this schema impacts other cognitions and as well as attitudes, cognitive-processing skills, and automatic thoughts (Renner et al., 2013). In this diathesis–stress model of depression, this schema is believed to be a crucial vulnerability for risk of depression (Ingram, Miranda, & Segal, 1998).

Case conceptualization is important in CBT for PDD and may focus more on modifying EMSs

The goal of CBT and schema-based therapies is to identify and modify these schemas in order to facilitate change and improve mood and functioning (Moore & Garland, 2003). When addressing PDD, there may be an increased focus on specific core beliefs and schemas that impact low self-esteem, helplessness, and hopelessness. These are often EMSs, which are entrenched, rigid, and overgeneralized negative core beliefs. It is helpful to describe the effects of these negative beliefs on the mood and behaviors of the patient and also to link them to the chronicity of depression. These typically take the form of unlovable, defective, incompetent, mistrustful, dependence, or abandonment schemas. The therapist and patient then collaborate to identify targets that will help challenge these schemas and combat these beliefs.

Specific goals for treatment are explicitly determined in the initial part of CBT for PDD. CBT researchers and clinicians propose that it is important to help set goals with the patient so that achievement of the goals will help improve self-esteem and address helplessness and hopelessness (Moore & Garland, 2003; Renner et al., 2013). Additional maintaining factors, which are explored further in schema therapy, may include such things as interpersonal avoidance behaviors, nonassertive behaviors, and other dysfunctional coping (Renner et al., 2013). This information is incorporated into a case formulation or conceptualization of the PDD patient with a plan of action for treatment. CBT formulations are based on CBT work by Beck (2011), Persons (1989), and Moore and Garland (2003), and schema therapy work by Renner et al. (2013).

Specific achievable goals for treatment are explicitly determined in the initial part of CBT for PDD

CBT Mechanisms of Action

The cognitive theory of depression proposes that through formative developmental experiences, people acquire stable cognitive schemas reflecting dysfunctional beliefs or schemas about the self, the world, and the future (Beck, 1987). These beliefs or schemas may lie dormant until they are activated by relevant stressful life events. When activated, these schemas are hypothesized to predispose the individual to engage in maladaptive information-processing styles or errors in thinking that precipitate depressed mood and lead to depressive behaviors that serve to maintain negative mood in a self-perpetuating feedback loop, ultimately leading to PDD. The assumption is that changing the thinking (schemas) of a depressed patient is a central mechanism of CBT that leads to symptomatic relief (Beck, 1987). Cognitive therapists believe modifying the dysfunctional thinking that has perpetuated depressive symptoms will facilitate therapeutic change, by enabling modification of core cognitive schemas. Thus, cognitive interventions are considered the active ingredients of change. This is referred to as the **cognitive mediation hypothesis** (Beck, 1987). There have been a variety of models describing how this is presumed to happen. These models include the idea that CBT leads to cognitive change on a schema level, and this schema change removes underlying vulnerability emanating from the previously held maladaptive schemas. Another model proposes that CBT only deactivates the schemas temporarily, and that the underlying maladaptive schemas will return eventually under stress. There is also a model that advances the idea that newly formed functional schemas compete with old maladaptive schemas when the individual is under stress. Finally, there is a model that proposes that CBT does not change schemas at all but teaches patients to use compensatory skills that effectively help them improve their symptoms (Padesky, 1994).

Schemas are formed through formative developmental experiences and activated by current life events

Cognitive mediation hypothesis is that cognitive interventions are active ingredients of change in CBT

Unfortunately, the limited research to date has not produced consistent evidence that CBT produces any more change in measures of these variables than treatment with pharmacotherapy. Scott et al. (2000) conducted a study of CBT for patients with MDD and residual symptoms and explored the impact on relapse prevention. Specifically, these researchers explored whether the effects of CBT in preventing relapse were mediated by a number of cognitive

Modifying dysfunctional thinking is a proposed mechanism of action of CBT, but there is little support for this

measures, including dysfunctional attitudes, attributional style, and meta-awareness. CBT produced specific improvements in key symptoms of hopelessness and self-esteem. Consistent with previous studies, however, scores on measures of depression-related cognition provided no evidence that depressive symptoms were impacted by changes in the content of cognition (Scott et al., 2000).

Scott et al. (2000) created a measure of extreme responding on the questionnaires, and this measure did appear to mediate the relapse prevention effects of CBT. Extreme responding (endorsing primarily "totally agree" or "totally disagree") significantly predicted relapse in the sample as a whole and statistically accounted for the effects of CBT on depressive symptoms. Interestingly, the extremity measure included extreme positive as well as extreme negative responses. The researchers report that this suggests that the CBT worked by reducing absolute, dichotomous thinking style rather than simply by reducing negative cognitions. These researchers found that when they explored their measure of meta-awareness or the sense of thoughts as thoughts, rather than reality, they found that meta-awareness scores mediated the relapse prevention effects of CBT (Scott et al., 2000). Preventing relapse in patients with residual symptoms is not the same as treating active PDD patients, but this study does highlight potential mechanisms of action of CBT in addressing depression. Scott and colleagues (2000) concluded that the mechanism of action of CBT might be the change in thinking style, such that instead of emotionally relevant information being processed automatically in a dichotomous fashion, CBT helps change to a mode where emotional information can be held in awareness and responded to in a more intentional or mindful manner.

Changing thinking style instead of content may be the mechanism of action in CBT

CBT Efficacy and Prognosis

CBT has been well studied for acute or episodic depression, but less so for PDD. Early pilot studies on CBT in chronic MDD, DD, or double depression found inconsistent results. Agosti and Ocepek-Welikson (1997) compared the effectiveness of CBT, IPT, imipramine, and placebo clinical management (PCM) for outpatients with early-onset chronic depression ($N = 65$) in the National Institute of Mental Health (NIMH) Treatment of Depression Collaborative Research Program (TDRP). They found that the posttreatment depression scores of the CBT, IPT, and imipramine groups were not significantly different from those of the PCM group. These researchers reported a 50% drop in depression severity at posttreatment, measured by the HDRS, across all treatments, but patients remained significantly depressed at the end of treatment. They reported no significant relationship between the duration of MDD and response to a specific treatment (Agosti & Ocepek-Welikson, 1997).

Gloaguen, Cottraux, Cucherat, and Blackburn (1998) conducted a meta-analysis of CBT and other psychotherapies for MDD and DD, and concluded CBT was superior to "other therapies," which were defined as psychotherapies without distinct cognitive or behavioral components. However, they also found that the effects produced by the CBT versus other therapies comparisons were heterogeneous, indicating that some aspect of these comparisons was creating unexplained variance in the outcomes. Wampold, Minami, Baskin, and Callen Tierney (2002) reanalyzed this meta-analysis of the 22 RCTs comparing psychotherapies intended to be therapeutic for MDD and DD (interpersonal,

CBT and other psychotherapies have been found to be equally effective with a small effect size

insight-oriented, supportive, brief psychodynamic, relaxation) with CBT and found that all were equally efficacious, with a small effect size ($d+ = 0.16$).

However, in a review of meta-analyses, Hoffman, Asnaani, Vonk, Sawyer, and Fang (2012) summarized research on CBT for depression and DD and found that CBT was more effective than control conditions such as waitlist and relaxation, or no treatment, with an overall medium effect size. Additionally, Tolin (2010) showed CBT to be superior to psychodynamic therapy at both posttreatment and 6-month follow-up, although this occurred when depression and anxiety symptoms were examined together, and it is unclear if the depressive symptoms were chronic.

Hollon et al. (2016) investigated a subgroup of 159 patients with MDD who were randomly assigned to CBT plus pharmacotherapy or to pharmacotherapy alone, and reported that combined treatment enhanced the rate of recovery when compared with medication alone, 75.2% versus 65.6%; $t_{451} = 2.44$; $p = .02$; hazard ratio (HR) = 1.32; 95% CI, 1.06–1.65; NNT = 11; 95% CI, 6–91. This effect was limited to patients with severe but nonchronic MDD: 84.7% versus 57.7%; $n = 147$; $t_{146} = 3.88$; $p = .001$; HR = 2.21; 95% CI, 1.48–3.31; NNT = 4; 95% CI, 2–8.

Booster or maintenance sessions of CBT have been demonstrated to have a substantial effect on lowering the recurrence of depression in chronic patients who were CBT responders (Fava, Rafanelli, Grandi, Conti, & Belluardo, 1998). Jarrett et al. (2001) conducted a maintenance CBT study with patients suffering from chronic recurrent MDD and found that over an 8-month period, CBT significantly reduced relapse rates more than a control intervention (10% vs. 31% relapse, respectively).

> **Booster sessions of CBT may help prevent relapse**

4.1.3 Cognitive Behavioral Analysis System of Psychotherapy

CBASP was designed to address the entrenched interpersonal problems and maladaptive cognitive behavioral patterns that are so often found in PDD patients (McCullough, 2000). The CBASP theory proposes that early interpersonal trauma or repeated psychological insults result in a learned lack of emotional felt safety, which leads to avoidance; derailed affective, social, and motivational regulation; and impaired **perceived functionality**. Perceived functionality is described as the ability to recognize the consequences of one's own behavior on other individuals and develop social problem-solving skills and empathy to achieve one's predetermined realistic and attainable interpersonal goals (McCullough, 2000; McCullough et al., 2015).

> **CBASP is specifically for early-onset unipolar chronic depression and is especially effective for patients with trauma histories**

The CBASP theory posits that PDD patients enter therapy dominated by interpersonal rigidity, and they are stuck in unproductive interactions because the current environment is not informing them. Specifically, the CBASP approach theorizes that the depressed patient does not grasp their contribution to the life difficulties they encounter, and that therapeutic strategies that rely on rational disputation, as in cognitive therapy, will not be effective with these PDD patients. The primary goal of CBASP is to enable patients to interact with greater interpersonal flexibility and to generate empathy for the therapist and eventually for others. This is achieved by increasing felt emotional safety

> **Primary goals of CBASP: to increase felt emotional safety and perceived functionality in PDD patients**

of the patient and facilitating more effective connection with the environment – that is, increasing the patient's perceived functionality. The CBASP approach is different from other therapies in that it explicitly describes the necessity of the therapist becoming involved as a representative of the social-emotional environment to facilitate learning, early in the therapeutic process with patients who have a paucity of interpersonal relationships or skills (McCullough, 2006).

One of the goals of CBASP is to help the patient gain the ability to recognize the interpersonal consequences of their behavior to be able to do the work of change. CBASP has demonstrated effectiveness in treating PDD and is also well-suited for patients who have extensive avoidance learning, high rates of early trauma, or repeated interpersonal failures, or who cope by "escaping," "avoiding," or "numbing" (Locke et al., 2017; Nemeroff et al., 2003). The phases of treatment and associated work to be done in CBASP for PDD are summarized in Box 3 and are compiled from McCullough and his colleagues (McCullough, 2000, 2006; McCullough et al., 2015).

Box 3
Stages of CBASP for Persistent Depressive Disorder

Assessment

- Therapist conducts a clinical or diagnostic assessment to determine presence of persistent depressive disorder (PDD) and other symptoms or diagnoses, with focus on clinical course over time.
- Severity of depression is assessed, as is suitability for cognitive behavioral analysis system of psychotherapy (CBASP).
- If patient is deemed suitable for CBASP, the therapist socializes the patient to CBASP and provides the Patient's Manual for CBASP (McCullough, 2003).
- Patient is asked to generate a list of significant individuals who have played a decisive and influential role in their life, and to bring it for the next session. This list should be fairly short with about three to five individuals listed. The patient is encouraged only to write down the names and not to think too hard about this exercise.

Initial sessions

- Therapist reviews the Patient's Manual with the patient and answers additional questions about CBASP.
- Therapist describes the rationale for the significant other history (SOH) and elicits the SOH from the list provided by the patient. Therapist formulates the causal theory conclusions from the SOH with the patient and also develops the transference hypothesis, which may or may not be shared with the patient.
- Therapist assesses the interpersonal impact of patient on the therapist via the Impact Message Inventory (IMI) or similar tool.

Middle sessions

- IMI is reviewed by therapist to help inform the therapist of the patient's interpersonal "stimulus values" to help define therapist's interpersonal role with the patient and any potential interpersonal "hot spots."
- Therapist orients the patient to the mainstay of CBASP – the situational analysis (SA) of the Coping Survey Questionnaire.
- Therapist conducts elicitation phase and remediation phase of the SAs during sessions, based on past or future events brought by the patient.

- Review and remediation of SAs is the focus of the majority of the time devoted, and the active treatment stage of therapy can last for 20 sessions or more.
- Patients are encouraged to continue with SA until they begin to formulate and achieve realistic and attainable interpersonal goals on their own, thus achieving perceived functionality.
- It is recommended that the patient be able eventually to successfully complete SAs on their own in session, thus demonstrating learning and transfer of learning.
- Therapist also uses the relationship with the patient to help modify patient behavior using disciplined personal involvement tools.
- Interpersonal discrimination exercises (IDEs) are used to help discriminate hurtful or threatening responses from people in the patient's life, from the helpful and supportive responses of the therapist, and explore the opportunities these insights afford the patient.
- Contingent personal responsivity (CPR): Contingent interpersonal reactions from the therapist toward the patient are used to target maladaptive behavior of the patient that interferes with the administration of CBASP. The CPR reaction from the therapist makes explicit the consequences of the patient's behavior on the clinician, with the goal of modifying the problem behavior of the patient.
- Patient acquisition learning is assessed regarding learning how to do the SA and discrimination learning between hurtful others and the therapist.

Termination and conclusion of acute treatment

- The essential goal of CBASP is for patients to learn to self-administer SA correctly. Thus, performance learning criterion must be achieved to terminate treatment. This is assessed via the Patient Performance Rating Form (PPRF). Assessed symptoms and functioning (presumably mediated by the above learning) should be significantly improved, and ideally the patient should be treated up to the point of remission, prior to termination.

Maintenance

- Continuation of treatment with scheduled booster sessions at longer intervals or as needed is recommended to help maintain gains and prevent relapse. This is again solidly based on learning theory and the idea that relapses occur when learning is not maintained and the patient reverts to old patterns of behavior.

CBASP Assessment

The assessment phase of CBASP involves a detailed diagnostic interview and assessment to determine appropriateness of the patient for treatment. This takes about 1–3 sessions to accomplish. The CBASP therapist will also focus on making an accurate diagnosis and developing with the patient a detailed clinical course of their symptoms over time using the TCGS (McCullough et al., 2016b). If the patient is assessed to be appropriate for CBASP, the therapist will orient the patient to the CBASP approach and collect additional information.

In CBASP, the therapist needs to focus on understanding the patient's particular psychopathology and developing a disciplined plan for assisting the patient in overthrowing their cycle of depression. Specifically, in the first sessions of CBASP, the therapist assesses the patient's motivation to change as well as their sense of helplessness and hopelessness, with the understanding that patients are perceptually disconnected from the idea that their behavior has consequences. The therapist assesses any therapy interfering behaviors

Assessment phase of CBASP includes making a diagnosis of PDD and its clinical course

that the patient demonstrates. These are conceptualized as learned avoidance behaviors with consequential interpersonal impacts, of which the patient is unaware, but the therapist must be aware and address during treatment.

Therapy interfering behaviors may include demonstrating profound avoidance or withdrawal behaviors with the therapist (e.g., not looking at the therapist, not speaking), or behaving in a consistently provocative, exceedingly hostile, or passive aggressive manner with the therapist. The therapist would note these behaviors and use them to inform the case formulation and the IMI (Kiesler & Schmidt, 2006) that they complete regarding the patient in the initial sessions. The IMI (see Section 1.7.4: Scales Assessing Constructs Related to PDD) is an assessment of the interpersonal impact of the patient on the therapist, which is assumed to reflect the impact of the patient on others in their interpersonal environment. The therapist also assesses if the patient is profoundly lacking in interpersonal interactions, and the therapist may initiate activity monitoring and scheduling to facilitate behavioral activation and engagement if needed.

The CBASP therapist provides the patient with the *Patient's Manual for CBASP* (McCullough, 2002), which helps to further orient the patient to therapy and provides written information about the rational and process of CBASP. Finally, the therapist introduces the two phases of CBASP (assessment and treatment) and the initial assignment for the patient, which is to generate a list of people who have played a decisive role in influencing the patient and shaping who the patient has become. These people are typically individuals who raised the patient or who significantly influenced the patient, either in a positive or negative fashion. Patients are asked to bring a list of between three and five names when they return for the next session.

CBASP Initial Sessions

The initial sessions following intake and assessment involve reviewing the patient manual and answering the patient's questions. CBASP is presented as a different kind of therapy than the patient may have experienced. The main work of the initial sessions is to obtain information regarding the impact of significant others using the significant other history (SOH) format. The purpose of the SOH is to lead to the development of the patient's **causal theory conclusions** and establishment of the **transference hypothesis** (TH) formulation and begin the treatment formulation. Elicitation of the SOH involves reviewing with patients their lists of significant others in a very structured manner to help define past learning and the impact on current interpersonal functioning. The specific structure for this verbal elicitation process is provided in Appendix 1 CBASP Significant Other History: Guide for Elicitation.

CBASP therapeutic work is informed by the transference hypothesis and interpersonal impact of the patient

Reviewing the SOH with the patient can take time and is often an emotional experience for patients, especially if they have not shared such information recently. The therapist should take the time to do this process slowly and respectfully and should also reassure the patient as to why this process is necessary. Increased affect is, however, desired and should not be avoided. The therapist remains supportive and lets the patient express affect in a safe way, and then describes how CBASP will help the patient learn to live intentionally, effectively, and happily. This is an intentional component of CBASP utilizing negative reinforcement with patients who have learned mistakenly that their depression is endless and unchanging.

From the causal theory conclusions, the THs can be formulated. These hypotheses are "if-then" statements that pinpoint the prominent trauma domains that result in anxiety, fear, or pain for the patient. One primary hypothesis is generated from the SOH causal theory conclusions – typically the most salient or relevant one. This hypothesis takes the form of a statement such as "If I get close to Dr. Penberthy, she will hurt me." Typically, the hypothesis will fall within one of four domains: intimacy, personal disclosure, making mistakes, and feeling or expressing negative emotions. TH examples for each of these domains are in Box 4. The TH content is utilized throughout treatment via the implementation of the interpersonal discrimination exercise (IDE). The goal of the IDE is to modify refractory trauma emotions by teaching patients to explicitly discriminate emotionally between the relationship with the psychotherapist and relationships with malevolent significant others who have hurt the individual. The underlying rationale for targeting a TH is based on a transfer-of-learning assumption that patients will transfer onto the therapist the interpersonal expectancies (both positive and negative) acquired from earlier learning with important individuals. The therapist relationship and work with the patient are informed by the generated hypothesis from the patient's developmental interpersonal history.

The goal of the interpersonal discrimination exercises is to help increase felt emotional safety

---

Box 4
Examples of CBASP Transference Hypotheses in Four Interpersonal Domains

Intimacy:
"If I get emotionally close to Dr. Penberthy, then she will hurt me."

Disclosure of need:
"If I disclose personal matters or needs to Dr. Penberthy, then she will use it against me and humiliate me."

Making mistakes:
"If I make a mistake while working with Dr. Penberthy, then she will berate and reject me."

Expression of negative affect:
"If I experience negative feelings toward or while with Dr. Penberthy, then she will punish me or abandon me."

Based on unpublished material by James P. McCullough, Jr., 2018.

The therapist also completes the IMI (Kiesler & Schmidt, 2006) and uses this information to help better understand the interpersonal pulls of being around the patient. The purpose of using the IMI in CBASP is to give the therapist further information that will guide the choices and plan of treatment. After the initial sessions, the therapist completes the IMI based on interactions with the patient. The tool is scored to create a profile on the circumplex, which provides information about the interpersonal impact of the patient on the therapist. This is likely to be representative of the patient's interpersonal impact on many other individuals in their life. The IMI data are not necessarily shared with the patient, although information about the interpersonal theory behind the IMI is shared. The scores on the IMI do not reflect how the therapist behaves toward the patient, but instead reflect how the therapist *feels* like behaving toward the patient. These feelings are probably similar to those experienced by most people who come in contact with the patient.

The IMI is used in CBASP to help inform the therapist of interpersonal "hot spots" with patient

The IMI consists of 56 questions and produces a type of conceptual stimulus value map graphically describing the covert reactions that one person "pulls" from another. When scored, it generates numbers that are placed around an interpersonal circumplex, reflecting these emotional and behavioral pulls within the therapist. The circumplex is divided into two universal, pervasive dimensions of interpersonal interactions which each have their own continuums: control or agency (continuum between *dominant* and *submissive*) and affiliation (continuum between *friendly*/approach and *hostile*/avoid). These dimensions can be represented graphically on a circle with eight equally spaced points representing the opposite poles of each dimension, and distance from center representing position along the continuum (*dominance* and *submissiveness* for control, and *friendliness* and *hostility* for affiliation), along with alternating adjacent combinations of these behaviors, including *friendly–dominant, friendly–submissive, hostile–submissive*, and *hostile–dominant*.

The therapist's role is designed on the basis of combined information from the TH and the IMI. The knowledge from the IMI allows the therapist to be more fully aware of the interpersonal "pulls" when interacting with the patient and to be not only mindful of them (e.g., aware that perceiving the patient as hostile–submissive will elicit the complimentary tendency of hostile–dominant in the therapist) but actively monitoring them and using that knowledge to guide interactions in order to avoid interpersonal pitfalls (McCullough, 2006). Additionally, knowledge of the TH can help inform the therapist regarding their role with the patient and can predict potential problematic interpersonal areas, thus allowing the therapist to be on the alert for such interactions and assumptions.

An example of a typical IMI circumplex completed by a CBASP therapist in response to interacting with a PDD patient can be found in Figure 3 – again, keeping in mind that the scores reflect pulls that the patient most likely elicits from others in addition to the therapist, Figure 3 shows the results of an IMI completed by the therapist in response to a fictitious PDD patient at the beginning of CBASP and after 20 sessions of CBASP. What this figure illustrates is what is commonly found in the research literature: PDD patients are typically submissive, withdrawn, and often perceived as hostile and hostile–submissive interpersonally, and thus, they often draw complementary hostile and hostile–dominant interpersonal responses from others (Locke et al., 2017; Locke, Sayegh, Weber, & Turecki, 2016).

The CBASP therapist finishes this phase of treatment by developing a case formulation that incorporates the SOH, TH, and IMI to help the therapist understand and counter the learned emotional fear and avoidance behaviors of the patient. A treatment plan is then generated based on the case formulation. Swan, Leibing-Wilson, MacVicar, and Sloan (2016) have formalized the approach in a case formulation diagram that encompasses all elements and allows expansion for incorporating comorbidities (Penberthy et al., 2017). This CBASP formulation incorporates key problems in living, a timeline of the disorder with onset and fluctuations of symptoms related to or triggered by life

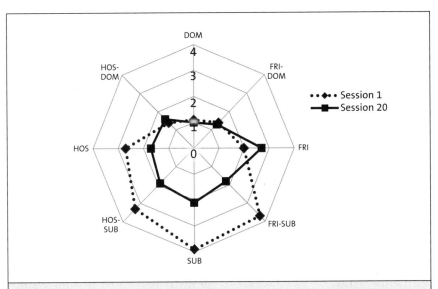

Figure 3

Impact Message Inventory scoring for a persistent depressive disorder (PDD) patient at Sessions 1 and 20 of cognitive behavioral analysis system of psychotherapy (CBASP) treatment. PDD patient initially elicits primarily submissive, friendly–submissive, hostile–submissive, and hostile interpersonal responses from others. Over time, with 20 sessions of CBASP, the patient's interpersonal style has changed to elicit friendlier and less submissive and hostile pulls. DOM = dominant; FRI-DOM = friendly–dominant; FRI = friendly; FRI-SUB = friendly–submissive; SUB = submissive; HOS-SUB = hostile–submissive; HOS = hostile; HOS-DOM = hostile–dominant.

events, the impact of significant others on interpersonal learning (including the causal theory conclusion and TH of the patient), and the current interpersonal profile of the patient, as well as a description of the actual problematic interpersonal behaviors and plans for exploring the consequence of those for the therapist and in the larger environment. An example of a CBASP case formulation worksheet for a fictitious PDD patient, Allison D., can be found in Appendix 2, and a blank worksheet can be found in Appendix 3.

CBASP Middle Sessions

Situational analysis (SA) of the Coping Survey Questionnaire (CSQ) is the core technique used during the middle sessions of CBASP and is based on the works of McCullough (2000, 2006) and colleagues (McCullough et al., 2015). This is an interpersonal problem-solving tool that helps the patient actively re-experience an interpersonal encounter and safely learn social-emotional interpersonal problem-solving skills. It is a step-wise process involving elicitation and remediation phases (Box 3). The therapist introduces the patient to the concept of SA and goes through the steps with the patient (see Appendix 4 CBASP Situational Analysis Format for the Coping Survey Questionnaire). SA is taught to the patient as a social problem-solving algorithm that has several interrelated aims: to expose and modify discrete maladaptive thoughts and behaviors, to promote awareness of the consequences of thoughts and

SA of a completed CSQ is an interpersonal problem-solving tool used during CBASP

behaviors, and to identify and change depression-maintaining patterns. These exercises help patients form causal connections between their mood symptoms and behaviors, which ultimately help in undoing these patterns. An example of an SA elicitation form is a found in Appendix 5 Elicitation Phase Prompts for Situational Analysis in CBASP.

The patient is asked to monitor distressing events that occur between sessions and record them on the form. Typically, patients focus on interpersonal events, but other events can also be targeted (e.g., the patient's avoidance of tasks). In each session, only one event is targeted and, within that event, the most meaningful slice of time (i.e., a starting point and ending point). There are three components to doing the SA: the elicitation phase, the remediation phase, and generalization. During the elicitation phase, the patient is encouraged to review the event according to its different components – namely: a description of the observable aspects of the event (as if they were watching a movie clip); the patient's main "reads" ("meaning statements") and thoughts or interpretations of the situation; the patient's behaviors and actions; the **actual outcome** (AO) in observable and behavioral terms; and the **desired outcome** (DO) in observable and behavioral terms. Patients are asked whether their AOs equaled their DOs. They are then asked why or why not this was so. These questions are meant to challenge the preoperational patient and should not be skipped. This maneuver sets the stage for the patient to see how they play an active role in affecting distressing interpersonal outcomes and may also enhance affect, which will be effectively addressed during the remediation phase of the exercise, thus employing negative reinforcement to help address the patient's helplessness and hopelessness.

The remediation phase is the next step in the SA process. The outline for remediation and suggested terminology is found in Appendix 6. The therapist helps the patient examine the situation and outcomes by exploring the role of the patient. If the therapist has determined that the DO was not achieved, because it is not realistic or attainable, meaning either the patient is not capable of producing it or the environment cannot produce it, the therapist should use Socratic questioning to gauge the patient's understanding of the DO. When necessary the therapist may wonder aloud if the DO is a realistic and achievable goal. This is done with a gentle curiosity similar to a motivational interviewing style of questioning. The patient is encouraged to conceptualize DOs as necessarily needing to be realistic and attainable and is urged to think of an acceptable DO if needed. The DO will need to be revised until it is an attainable and realistic one, as judged by the therapist and patient together. The therapist is encouraged to let the patient come to this determination of a realistic and attainable DO. Patients may struggle, but it will mean more if they determine themselves that the goals they have set are not feasible and work to modify them. Therapists are encouraged not to rush the process, but instead slow it to the pace of the patient and pay attention to the interpersonal pulls. The optimal interpersonal place for a CBASP therapist to be is in the friendly, friendly–dominant, and friendly–submission quadrants. Above all, CBASP therapists must act with awareness of their own intentions and be flexible in their interpersonal approach.

When a realistic, attainable goal is set, the therapist can proceed to the remediation phase. One primary goal is to help the patient learn to evaluate something during a concise period of time with a beginning, middle, and end. This is often challenging for PDD patients, as they are accustomed to thinking and talking globally and vaguely. Having the patient describe the "slices of time" can be helpful and is a kind of mindfulness exercise in itself, compelling the patient to narrow their attention and describe in a nonjudgmental way the unfolding of events. The therapist then focuses on connecting the interpretations and behaviors of the patient to facilitate the DO. This is done in a methodical, step-wise fashion by asking the patient a series of questions about their thoughts, judgments, and reading of the situation just described. The patient is asked if each of these interpretations is relevant to the DO, is accurate in its description, and if it contributes toward achieving the DO. The interpretations and behaviors are reviewed in turn, with the patient and therapist jointly determining if the interpretations or behaviors are relevant, accurate, or neither.

The next step is to provide an opportunity for the patient to revise the interpretations and/or behaviors in favor of ones that may be more consistent with the DO. This may involve helping the patient to revise interpretations, generate new action-oriented interpretations of the situation, or add assertive or friendly behaviors to their repertoire. Additional behavioral training such as assertiveness training or anger management can take place at the end of sessions in skills-training segments of therapy.

After all interpretations and behaviors of the patient have been reviewed, their impact on the DO evaluated, the interpretations and behaviors revised or adjusted, with any action interpretations added, the therapist asks the patient, if they had thought in this revised way and behaved in the new way, would they have achieved the DO? This question is rhetorical but meant to help underscore learning. The generalization phase of CBASP includes asking the patient what they have learned from going through the SA. The therapist also asks the patient to explicitly generalize, by asking if there are other situations where this new learning could be applied.

The administration of **disciplined personal involvement** (DPI) is the third component of the CBASP approach (see Box 3) and is interwoven throughout the sessions (McCullough, 2000, 2006). These techniques utilize data from the TH and IMI within the review of SAs in real time in a contingent and intentional manner to help the patient increase felt emotional safety and learn to discriminate between past negative responses by hurtful others, and positive and supportive responses from the CBASP therapist. PDD patients typically evoke several interpersonal reactions from individuals with whom they interact – these responses often include hostile and dominant behavior that frequently puts patients in a submissive interpersonal position. When clinicians don't engage in these destructive interpersonal strategies or when therapists respond to patients in a complementary or interpersonal manner unexpected by the patient due to their learning history, patients are given the opportunity to learn more adaptive interpersonal behavior in a safe interpersonal environment.

There are two techniques for implementing disciplined personal involvement in CBASP: **contingent personal responsivity** (CPR) and IDEs (McCullough, 2000, 2006) (for IDEs, see also the section "CBASP Initial Sessions"). The goals of these exercises are to demonstrate to the patient that their behavior has consequences, and to heal refractory trauma emotionality

DPI is used in CBASP to help facilitate felt emotional safety in the PDD patient

Two techniques for implementing disciplined personal involvement in CBASP are CPR and IDEs

by teaching the patient to discriminate between the therapist and malevolent significant others. CBASP's basic motif is to connect the patient perceptually to their current environment in an accurate and meaningful way.

CPR is used in CBASP to help the patient understand his or her interpersonal impact on the therapist

The first way disciplined personal involvement is used in CBASP is in instances where the therapist clarifies the consequences of the behavior of the patient by disclosing personal reactions and feelings produced by the behavior of the patient. This is what is meant by CPR (McCullough, 2006). The goals of this exercise are to teach the patient that they have an impact on others in their environment, including the therapist; to modify hurtful behaviors of the patient; and to transfer new interpersonal skills to other relationships outside of therapy. Several caveats of this exercise are that the personal reaction of the therapist must be explicitly pinpointed for the patient; the specific behavior that pulled the reaction must be identified; and the patient must be shown explicitly that the effect on the therapist derives from the connection. When used appropriately, the patient can be made aware of their impact on others and how this impacts their interpersonal interactions.

Clinical Vignette 1

CBASP IDE Administration Prompt Guidelines and Example

The CBASP interpersonal discrimination exercise (IDE) step-procedure based on the transference hypothesis (TH):

Step 1: The IDE can be administered whenever a patient and therapist start to talk about material or participate in an in-session event that is related to the identified patient TH.

For example, if the patient's identified TH is *"If I let Dr. P. get emotionally close to me, she will abandon or hurt me,"* and the patient has just disclosed something they feel emotionally vulnerable about and is now crying, this would be a good time to use an IDE.

Step 2: Therapist administers IDEs by asking several questions of the patient in a warm, curious, and gentle interpersonal style:

Therapist: Allison, what would your father have done if you shared with him what you just shared with me? And if you cried in front of him?

Allison: He would not have put up with it, and told me to shut up.

Therapist: Yes, I believe you are correct, that is what he would have done. Let me ask you, how did I react to you just now?

Allison: You were kind and understanding.... You listened to me.

Therapist: What are the *differences* between his reaction in the past and mine just now? What is different about *what* you experienced then, and *what* you have just experienced with me?

Allison: He would have rejected me and told me I am stupid. You listened and understood. You were kind and helpful.

Therapist: What are the interpersonal implications *for you*, if I respond differently to you in this situation? What does that mean for you?

Allison: I am not sure. I know this feels better and safer.... I guess maybe there is some hope.

IDEs help the patient modify refractory negative emotions

The second DPI technique is the use of IDEs, which are a Pavlovian emotional retraining exercise. A template for using IDEs and an example with a fictitious patient, Allison D., can be found in Clinical Vignette 1. The idea of an IDE is to catch the patient in a situation where the therapist is reacting to them in a very different and more productive way than hurtful others did in the past, and point this out to them. Then, the therapist discriminates themselves from the negative significant others by focusing the patient's attention on the differences between the therapist's behaviors in the trauma domain, compared explicitly with those of the traumatizing significant others.

An IDE is meant to modify refractory negative emotions associated with earlier trauma experiences. McCullough (2006) proposes that the perceptual disconnection existing between the patient and others, which is maintained through avoidance, perpetuates the depressed mood state, and the emotions remain refractory to change. The basic assumption of an IDE is that no emotional change is possible until the patient reconnects themselves to the original trauma event context and learns to feel emotional reactions other than fear, anxiety, or pain. The goals of IDE are for patients to experience novel ("safety") emotions in the context of the trauma or psychological insults domains (discussed in the SAs) that previously led to hurtful consequences and avoidance behavior; to awaken to a new awareness of interpersonal behavioral possibilities with the therapist; to identify individuals on the outside who will respond in a similar, salubrious fashion; and to learn to self-administer the IDE without assistance from the therapist.

Therapists who use DPI must be certain that they do not use these techniques in a punitive or demeaning manner to meet their own psychological needs. The disciplined component of the techniques mandates that the goal always be to facilitate learning in the patient (McCullough, 2006).

CBASP Conclusion of Acute Treatment

Patient acquisition learning is assessed throughout CBASP via standardized symptom measures and patient performance rating scales for the SA and IDE, as well as evaluations of percentage belief in the patient's TH over time. The goals of CBASP are clear and measureable, and learning acquisition is hypothesized to translate into increased felt emotional safety and learned perceived functionality (McCullough et al., 2015). These changes are hypothesized to impact mood and functioning positively in the PDD patient. These goals of treatment are determined collaboratively with the patient, and the patient is very aware of the criteria for concluding the acute phase of treatment. CBASP encourages that patients receive treatment until they are in full remission (McCullough, 2000). Studies to date have typically included 20–25 sessions of CBASP for the acute phase of treatment.

CBASP encourages patients to receive treatment until they are in full remission

CBASP Maintenance and Relapse Prevention

Sessions may be tapered toward the end of therapy if the patient has progressed, and strategies to help maintain learning are discussed with the patients prior to termination. Treatment may last for over a year, with follow-up maintenance sessions lasting for years. The CBASP therapist emphasizes that the learning achieved by the patient must be maintained, or relapse may occur. Thus, we encourage patients to continue the specific strategies they learned for living effectively. Situations or interactions that may increase the patient's vulnerability to relapse are reviewed, and strategies to maintain learning gains are reinforced. Booster sessions to help maintain learning and prevent relapse are recommended.

Ongoing maintenance or booster sessions are recommended in CBASP after end of treatment phase

CBASP Mechanisms of Action

CBASP mechanisms
may include
reducing fear and
avoidance and
increasing perceived
functionality

CBASP was designed to address the entrenched interpersonal problems and maladaptive cognitive behavioral patterns characteristic of PDD patients (McCullough, 2000). PDD is viewed as a mood disorder ensuing from biopsychosocial factors, driven by learned Pavlovian fears of interpersonal encounters, and maintained by a refractory pattern of Skinnerian interpersonal avoidance; as a result, a disconnect between the patient and the environment ensues. Thus, the CBASP approach is built upon the belief that effective treatment reduces symptomatology via cognitive, affective, and behavioral changes that enable patients to reduce interpersonal fear and avoidance, perceive the functionality of their behavior, reconnect to their environments, and increase their perception of control. The two primary goals of CBASP are (1) to quiet interpersonal fear and avoidance and replace it with felt emotional safety, and (2) to help patients acquire perceived functionality.

McCullough (2000, 2006) maintains that promoting felt emotional safety with the therapist is a necessary component for effective treatment. This mechanism can be assessed via a number of methods including ratings of interpersonal impact of the patient on the therapist over time or by measuring therapeutic alliance. Constantino et al. (2008) evaluated data from a large CBASP clinical trial and found that therapeutic alliance predicted decreases in patient hostile-submissiveness during therapy and significantly related to lower final session depression scores. They endorsed this as evidence that the increased felt emotional safety is a key mechanism of action in CBASP. However, more direct support for this hypothesized mechanism is currently lacking in the research literature.

Perceived functionality, which can be conceptualized as a form of social problem solving, is also hypothesized to be a mechanism of action for reducing depression in patients with PDD. Klein et al. (2011) explored the relationships among treatment, social problem solving, and depression in a randomized controlled trial (RCT) comparing CBASP with brief supportive psychotherapy (BSP) and pharmacotherapy. They found that CBASP plus pharmacotherapy was associated with significant improvement in social problem-solving skills versus BSP plus pharmacotherapy and that change in social problem solving predicted subsequent changes in depressive symptoms over time.

Santiago et al. (2005) explored the influences of therapeutic alliance (felt emotional safety) and ability to conduct the situational analysis (based on a patient performance rating scale for the situational analysis exercise in CBASP) on outcome measures of depression in a CBASP trail. Their findings confirmed that good initial alliances were associated with lower endpoint levels of depressive symptoms and that a better patient ability to perform an SA was associated with lower endpoint levels of depression. They found no mediating or moderating effects of therapeutic alliance via its impact on SA or vice versa, and thus concluded that the alliance and social problem-solving skills promoted change in PDD patients via separate mechanisms. There has been little additional research exploring the hypothesized mechanisms of action in CBASP, and no systematic dismantling research completed to date.

CBASP Efficacy and Prognosis

CBASP hit the scene in a big way with a large multicenter RCT of 681 chronically depressed patients at 12 sites across the US (Keller et al., 2000). This trial compared the effectiveness of 12 weeks of nefazodone alone, CBASP therapy alone, and the combination of both. Patients in the CBASP-alone and combined-treatment groups received 12–16 sessions of psychotherapy. Among the 519 participants who completed the study, the rates of response were 55% in the nefazodone group and 52% in the psychotherapy group, as compared with 85% in the combined-treatment group ($p < .001$ for both comparisons). The authors conclude that both of the monotherapies yielded similarly efficacious results, with no differences found between them ($g = 0.04$, $SE = 0.10$, 95% CI, –0.15 to 0.23, $p = .68$). The combination of CBASP and nefazodone was more effective in reducing symptoms than either CBASP alone ($g = 0.54$, $SE = 0.10$, 95% CI, 0.35–0.73, $p < .001$) or nefazodone alone ($g = 0.49$, $SE = 0.10$, 95% CI, 0.31–0.68, $p < .001$). The average effect size comparing the combined treatment with the monotherapies was $g = 0.52$ ($SE = 0.10$, 95% CI, 0.43–0.82, $p < .001$). The effects calculated from mean change scores produced an effect size of $g = 0.55$ ($SE = 0.10$, 95% CI 0.37–0.74, $p < .001$) for the comparison of combined treatment versus nefazodone alone, and for the comparison of combined treatment versus CBASP alone produced an effect size of $g = 0.64$ ($SE = 0.10$, 95% CI, 0.45–0.83, $p < .001$). A secondary analysis of the temporal sequence of symptom change showed that the overall advantage of the combined group was attributable to sharing both the earlier onset of benefit seen in the nefazodone-alone condition and the later-emerging benefit seen in the CBASP-alone condition (Keller et al., 2000).

The Keller et al. (2000) trial also implemented a crossover phase for nonresponders to monotherapies (61 patients in CBASP; 79 patients in nefazodone). Patients in both arms showed clinical benefits by switching so that at 24 weeks their outcomes matched those of the combined group at 12 weeks (Schatzberg et al., 2005). The study had a continuation phase, with 12 monthly sessions added to the acute treatment phase. In this continuation phase, 82 patients who had responded to CBASP were randomly assigned to either once-monthly CBASP sessions or assessment appointments. In the intent-to-treat sample, overall response rates were significantly higher for patients who crossed over to CBASP from nefazodone (57%; 35/61) than for patients who crossed over to nefazodone from CBASP (42%, 33/79; $\chi^2 = 5.03$, $p = .03$). In the CBASP condition, significantly fewer patients experienced recurrence than in the assessment-only condition (Klein et al., 2004).

Another CBASP trial (Kocsis et al., 2009) evaluated a total of 808 patients with chronic depression across eight academic sites. In the first phase of this study, participants received 12 weeks of open-label antidepressant medication according to a pharmacotherapy algorithm similar to that of the STAR*D study. In the second phase of the study, patients who had not responded or only partially responded to medication received all next-step pharmacotherapy options with or without adjunctive psychotherapy and were assigned to one of three treatment conditions for another 12 weeks: a medication switch or augmentation, supplementary CBASP, or supplementary supportive therapy (SPT) as active control condition. This study failed to find clear advantages of CBASP supplemented with medication over SPT ($g = 0.18$, $SE = 0.11$, 95%

CI, −0.04 to 0.39, $p = 0.10$) or antidepressant monotherapy ($g = 0.12$, $SE = 0.14$, 95% CI, −0.15 to 0.39, $p = .39$). Comparing the efficacy of CBASP with the average effect observed in the control groups (SPT, medication), a nonsignificant and small effect size resulted ($g = 0.15$, $SE = 0.13$, 95% CI, −0.10 to 0.41, $p = .24$). The effect sizes that were calculated from mean change scores of CBASP and SPT ($g = 0.16$, $SE = 0.08$, 95% CI, 0.01–0.31, $p = .04$) as well as for CBASP and medication only ($g = 0.28$, $SE = 0.10$, 95% CI, 0.09–0.48, $p = .004$) turned out to be small, but significant, respectively. These results should be interpreted with caution, however, because the study may have selected patients with a preference for drug treatment, and the number of therapy sessions was low.

Reviews and meta-analysis of RCTs of CBASP for PDD have concluded that CBASP is effective (Jobst et al., 2016; Negt et al., 2016). Specifically, Negt and colleagues (2016) evaluated six RCTs and assessed the efficacy of CBASP in PDD. A combined overall effect size of $g = 0.34$ ($SE = 0.13$, 95% CI 0.09–0.59, $p = .007$) was obtained. Compared with the control conditions, CBASP produced a significant combined effect size of small magnitude. To investigate more general efficacy of CBASP in PDD, a combined effect size was calculated ($g = 0.34$, $SE = 0.13$, 95% CI, 0.09–0.59, $p = .007$). The overall combined effect size obtained from mean change scores of CBASP and the comparison conditions was $g = 0.44$ ($SE = 0.07$, 95% CI, 0.31–0.57, $p < .001$, $Q = 5.11$, $I^2 = 2.14$, $p = .40$). Negt et al. (2016) concluded that the combined overall effect sizes of CBASP versus other treatments or treatment as usual (TAU) demonstrated a significant effect of small magnitude ($g = 0.34–0.44$, $p < .01$). The researchers further offer that CBASP demonstrated moderate-to-high effect sizes when compared with TAU and IPT ($g = 0.64–0.75$, $p < .05$), and showed trends toward similar effect sizes when compared with antidepressant medication alone ($g = –0.29$ to 0.02, ns). The combination of CBASP and antidepressant medication demonstrated benefits when compared with antidepressants only ($g = 0.49–0.59$, $p < .05$). Thus, CBASP in combination with pharmacotherapy was found to be more effective than CBASP alone. Based on a network meta-analysis comparing the efficacy and acceptability of several treatment approaches for chronic depression, Kriston, von Wolff, Westphal, Hölzel, and Härter (2014) reported that IPT was less effective than medication (OR = 0.48) and CBASP (OR = 0.45). Compared with the combined effect size from the Cuijpers, van Straten, et al. (2010) review of psychotherapy treatments for DD and chronic MDD ($d = 0.23$), the increased and significant combined effect size of CBASP studies in this same population ($g = 0.34–0.44$) is encouraging.

Jobst et al. (2016) also performed a systematic review of studies on psychotherapy for PDD and developed recommendations for treatment approaches based upon their findings. They presented their findings on IPT, CBT and CBASP among others and also included studies exploring pharmacotherapy alone or in addition to psychotherapy. Jobst et al. (2016) summarized findings from 35 studies (six meta-analyses and reviews, 18 RCTs, 11 cohort or open studies, case series) and developed five recommendations based on their findings. The first recommendation was regarding choice of psychotherapy. The methodology of each study was assessed to appraise its validity according to the recommendation-grading scheme of the Scottish Intercollegiate Guidelines

CBASP has a moderate-high effect size compared with IPT and pharmacotherapy

Combining CBASP with an effective antidepressant medication may increase effectiveness

Network (Scottish Intercollegiate Guidelines Network, 2011). They used the results of this assessment to determine the level of evidence for each study: Level 1++ (high-quality meta-analyses, systematic reviews with low risk of bias) to Level 4 (expert opinion). These levels of evidence were used to determine a recommendation grade (Grade A = *top rating*; Grade D = *lowest rating*). Jobst et al. (2016) endorsed CBASP and, to a lesser degree, IPT therapy as most effective as a first-line psychotherapy for PDD. Specifically, CBASP was recommended with an evidence level of 1++ or Grade A and IPT with an evidence level of 1 and Grade B. They recommended CBT as a third-line psychotherapy with an evidence level of 2+ and Grade C. Additional recommendations from Jobst and colleagues (2016) included providing personalized treatment to patients based on their preferences and ensuring that pharmacotherapy is provided at an adequate frequency and duration to help ensure effective "dosing" for the acute phase of treatment and continued in maintenance treatment.

Jobst et al. (2016) endorsed CBASP as a first line psychotherapy for PDD

Klein et al. (2004) have produced robust data suggesting that maintenance treatment with CBASP after termination of the initial treatment phase is effective in preventing recurrences. These researchers randomized patients who had responded to an intensive 12-week acute-phase course of CBASP and maintained their response through a 16- week continuation phase to 52 weeks of maintenance phase CBASP (with sessions conducted every 4 weeks) or assessment only. Recurrence was defined in the protocol as a HDRS score of 16 or greater on two consecutive visits, and a diagnosis of MDD as determined from a DSM-IV MDD checklist administered by an independent evaluator. Using the protocol definition, Kaplan-Meier product-limit estimates of the rates of recurrence were 2.6% in the CBASP condition compared with 20.9% in the assessment-only condition, log-rank test (1) 4.76, $p = .03$. Using the consensus definition, the researchers found estimated recurrence rates of 10.7% and 32.0% in the CBASP and assessment-only conditions, respectively, log-rank test (1) 3.99, $p = .05$. In both analyses, the protective effects of CBASP appeared to emerge after 5–6 months of maintenance treatment. The authors suggest that the benefits of maintenance CBASP may include continued reduction of subthreshold symptoms (Klein et al., 2004).

Maintenance CBASP is highly recommended and has been found to prevent recurrences of depression

McCullough et al. (2015) hypothesize that relapse or recurrence occurs when active reinforcers of treatment are withdrawn, and patients are effectively placed on an extinction schedule. Thus, ongoing practice on the part of the patient is imperative for continued remission from depression. This can be achieved through the use of specific self-monitoring and CBASP work by the patient alone, or preferably, with the CBASP psychotherapist as needed after the active treatment phase.

4.1.4 Mindfulness-Based Cognitive Therapy

There is a significant risk of relapse in patients with PDD, even in fully remitted individuals. In MDD, the risk of relapse increases with successive episodes experienced. Even among patients who achieve clinical remission, residual depressive symptoms (RDSs) following first-line antidepressant pharmacotherapy or psychotherapy are common (Hardeveld et al., 2013). Psychological

MBCT may be useful in preventing relapse in PDD

accounts of MDD vulnerability emphasize how state-dependent learning links the experience of dysthymia with self-evaluative and ruminative cognitive styles, with each MDD episode strengthening the elements of this cognitive-affective network. Over time, even mild levels of low or sad mood can trigger depressive cognitive thought patterns that lead to increased rates of depressive symptoms (Teasdale, Segal, & Williams, 1995). Thus, a goal of MBCT is to preemptively foster an awareness of, and ability to understand and influence, these cognitive processes.

MBCT is a manualized therapy that combines the attentional training of mindfulness meditation with the activation and psychoeducation elements of cognitive therapy for depression (Segal, Williams, & Teasdale, 2013). MBCT typically involves eight weekly group sessions along with daily home assignments. It teaches formal meditations (such as body scan and sitting meditations) and informal mindfulness practices (such as mindfulness of everyday activities). Session topics include such things as dealing with barriers, staying present, the idea that thoughts are not facts, and using what has been learned to deal with future moods. Patients are taught to become more aware of thoughts and feelings, and to relate to them from a perspective that sees them as *mental events*, rather than as aspects of the self or as accurate reflections of reality. The theory is based on the belief that by developing this more objective relationship with depression-related thoughts and feelings, the individual is able to prevent the escalation of negative-thinking patterns or rumination at times of potential relapse or recurrence.

> **MBCT encourages patients to relate to thoughts and feelings as mental events**

MBCT Mechanisms of Action

> **MBCT is hypothesized to work by increasing mindfulness and reducing ruminations**

MBCT was developed as a psychological intervention for preventing relapse in patients with a history of depressive disorders, including PDD. Hypothesized mechanisms of change for this intervention are in line with MBCT's theoretical underpinnings and include increases in mindfulness and/or decreases in negative repetitive thoughts or ruminations. Recent reviews (Gu, Strauss, Bond, & Cavanagh, 2015; van der Velden et al., 2015) have explored the mechanisms of change and demonstrated that both mindfulness and repetitive negative thoughts were significant mediators of the effect of MBCT on mental health outcomes, including anxiety, depressive symptoms, general psychopathology, stress, and negative affect. Both of these papers provided strong evidence that increased mindfulness and decreased negative repetitive thought (i.e., rumination) are processes that mediate the association among mindfulness-based interventions and treatment outcome.

MBCT Efficacy and Prognosis

> **MBCT may be added after other psychotherapies**

An 8-week RCT conducted in Germany (Michalak, Schultze, Heidenreich, & Schramm, 2015) examined the effects of group MBCT and TAU, group CBASP and TAU, and TAU alone, in 106 chronically depressed patients. All enrolled participants met the criteria for PDD (either chronic MDD and/or DD). The primary outcome measure was the HDRS score at the end of treatment. Secondary outcome measures were the BDI and measures of social functioning and quality of life. Remission was defined as a HDRS score of 8 or less at posttreatment. MBCT produced an effect size of $g = 0.42$ ($S = 0.05$, 95% CI, 0.33–0.52, $p < 0.001$) compared with TAU. CBASP led to a significantly greater decrease in HDRS scores than TAU, with the average change in CBASP participants being roughly 0.82 SDs larger than that of the TAU group ($p < .001$). The effect size comparing CBASP with the combined control condition (MBCT, TAU) was of small size and achieved marginal significance ($g = 0.41$, $SE = 0.24$, 95% CI, -0.06 to 0.88, $p = .09$). The mean change effect size comparing CBASP with TAU was $g = 0.71$ ($SE = 0.22$, 95% CI, 0.27–1.15, $p = .001$). The mean change effect of CBASP and MBCT yielded an effect size of $g = 0.23$ ($SE = 0.22$, CI, -0.15 to 0.70, $p = .20$) (Michalak et al., 2015).

Teasdale et al. (2000) have shown in two studies that training in MBCT can reduce risk of relapse or recurrence in patients initially treated with medications only. MBCT had its strongest preventive effects on patients with three or more prior episodes, a pattern of moderation that suggests that it may work through different mechanisms from standard CBT. A subsequent trial found MBCT to be more effective than maintenance medication in reducing residual depressive symptoms and in improving quality of life; 75% of the MBCT patients in that trial were able to discontinue medications (Kuyken et al., 2015). Differences in rates of relapse and recurrence favored MBCT but were not significant. Additional research is still required regarding MBCT, but it may be a helpful addition after treatment with one of the psychotherapies reviewed above, to help prevent relapse.

4.1.5   Pharmacotherapy

Pharmacotherapy is an important component of a comprehensive treatment approach for PDD. Most psychologists will not prescribe medications for their PDD patients, but a basic knowledge of pharmacotherapy and the underlying neurobiology may be helpful. It can be helpful to know when it is appropriate to refer for a pharmacotherapy evaluation and what to consider when making the referral. A referral may be appropriate when the patient's depression is so severe that meaningful participation in therapy is impossible. It might be advisable to refer when the clinician thinks that therapy would be augmented by a medication – for instance, if sleep, appetite, or energy are so severely impacted and psychotherapy has not helped significantly. Some patients will request pharmacotherapy. Many patients may need education about the effects and limitations of pharmacotherapy, and it is incumbent upon psychologists who are following such patients to educate themselves regarding these medications. The task of helping patients understand the role and limits of pharmacotherapy, how to maintain adherence, the positive and negative side effects, and limitations of pharmacotherapy often falls to the psychologist.

Overall, the choice of a specific antidepressant for PDD is typically the same as for more acute forms of depression. Antidepressants from various classes have been reported to be equally effective for the treatment of patients with various forms of PDD. Most studies in the research literature have included patients diagnosed with either DD or MDD, and few specify the classification of double depression or PDD. The primary differences between the antidepressants are their side effect profiles. Knowledge of symptoms of depression and potential underlying neurobiological components may help

Different antidepressant medications appear to be equally effective

psychiatrists or other physicians prescribe the most appropriate and effective pharmacotherapy. Saltiel and Silvershein (2015) propose a pharmacotherapeutic approach based on the treatment of select symptoms in MDD patients and include evaluating which medication to provide based on key presenting symptoms of anxiety, cognitive problems, insomnia, fatigue or low energy, pain, psychomotor problems, appetite problems, and sleepiness. Thus, the psychologist's assessment of these symptoms when referring for pharmacotherapy evaluation can be informative for physicians or other health professionals. It is also important to clarify with the patient any prior history of taking medications for depression or anxiety, whether these worked or not, and if there were any negative side effects. Any unresolved residual symptoms, treatment-emergent symptoms, and comorbid disorders need to be carefully assessed and incorporated into the formulation.

The earlier antidepressant mediations were the **tricyclics**, named thus because of their molecular structures which contain three rings of atoms (Table 10). These medications include imipramine, amitriptyline, and clomipramine, and work by increasing norepinephrine and serotonin and inhibiting their reuptake. A few of the tricyclics also influence dopamine. The challenge with these

Table 10
Antidepressant Medications and Trade Names

Medication	Trade Name
Tricyclics	
Amitriptyline	Elavil
Clomipramine	Anafranil
Desipramine	Norpramin
Doxepin	Sinequan
Imipramine	Tofranil
Nortriptyline	Pamelor
Trimipramine	Surmontil
SSRIs	
Citalopram	Celexa
Escitalopram	Lexapro
Fluoxetine	Prozac
Fluvoxamine	Luvox
Paroxetine	Paxil
Sertraline	Zoloft
SNRIs	
Duloxetine	Cymbalta
Venlafaxine	Effexor
Desvenlafaxine	Pristiq
Nefazodone	Serzone
NDRI	
Bupropion	Wellbutrin

Note. NDRI = norepinephrine-dopamine reuptake inhibitor; SNRIs = serotonin-norepinephrine reuptake inhibitor; SSRIs = selective serotonin reuptake inhibitor.

early medications is that, although they work in reducing depressive symptoms, they also cause negative side effects because they are not selective with respect to their neurobiological targets. Thus, tricyclics are typically not the first-line antidepressant for most patients with PDD but may be used if other antidepressants do not appear to work. Since the 1990s, a newer generation of antidepressants has been more widely available and has fewer side effects because their neurobiological targets are more selective. These commonly used antidepressants target the previously reviewed neurobiological components and include the **selective serotonin reuptake inhibitors** (SSRIs), **serotonin-norepinephrine reuptake inhibitors** (SNRIs), and **norepinephrine-dopamine reuptake inhibitors** (NDRIs) (Saltiel & Silvershein, 2015). A list of common antidepressant medications with their trade names can be found in Table 10.

> **Commonly prescribed medications for PDD include the SSRIs, SNRIs, and NDRIs**

Years of research have led to official guidelines for use of antidepressant medications. The APA has developed the most widely used guidelines, and they state that mediation is only one aspect of treatment of depression and that psychotherapy may be the most helpful treatment whether alone or in combination with pharmacotherapy (APA, 2010). These guidelines have suggestions regarding which medication to try first and what strategies to try if the first medication is not effective. Typically, an SSRI is started by the physician, and then after an adequate trial of the medication, if it is not tolerated or effective, the patient may be switched to an antidepressant of another class: for example, an SNRI or NDRI. Subsequent options include combination pharmacotherapy. As with psychotherapy, often the key to effective treatment is to give relatively high doses for relatively long periods of time.

> **Medication may be at higher doses for longer periods of time for PDD, compared with acute or episodic depression**
>
> **There are clinical guidelines regarding prescribing medication for depression**

Overall, the mechanisms of action of the tricyclics, SSRIs, SNRIs, and NDRIs are fairly well conceptualized and work about equally well for treating PDD (Linde, Kriston, et al., 2015). The medication response rate in PDD, though perhaps lower than that seen in acute MDD, is reproducibly higher than the placebo response rate (Kriston et al., 2014). Medication is significantly more effective than placebo in nearly all double-blind RCTs of DD (Fournier et al., 2010; Kriston et al., 2014).

> **Pharmacotherapy is significantly more effective than placebo**

4.2   Variations and Combinations of Methods

Clinical trials and research regarding treatment for PDD support providing psychotherapy combined with pharmacotherapy (Cuijpers, van Straten, et al., 2009, Cuijpers et al., 2014; Hollon et al., 2014; Jobst et al., 2016). In a meta-analysis of psychotherapy versus combination treatment for depression, Cuijpers, van Straten, et al. (2009) reviewed 18 studies ($N = 1,838$) and calculated effect sizes indicating the difference between psychotherapy only and combined treatments. An effect size of .8 was assumed to be large, whereas effect sizes of .5 were moderate, and effect sizes of .2 small. They found a mean effect size for the difference between psychotherapy and combined treatment of 0.35 (95% CI, 0.24–0.45; $p < .001$), with low heterogeneity. Cuijpers, van Straten, et al. (2009) also investigated 25 RCTs with 2,036 depressed patients and found a mean effect size of $d = 0.31$ (95% CI, 0.20–0.43), indicating a small effect in favor of the combined treatment over pharmacotherapy

> **Combining psychotherapy and pharmacotherapy may be more effective than either alone**

alone. Studies involving patients with DD resulted in significantly lower effect sizes compared with studies of patients with MDD, a finding that suggests that the added value of psychotherapy is attenuated in patients with DD. The researchers reported that the dropout rate was significantly lower in the combined-treatment group compared with the pharmacotherapy-only group (OR = 0.65, 95% CI, 0.50–0.83).

Cuijpers, Smit, et al. (2010) directly evaluated chronic MDD and DD in another meta-analysis of 16 studies with 2,116 patients. These studies included seven focused on CBT, six on IPT, and eight that were listed as "other therapies," including such things as problem-solving, cognitive–interpersonal, CBASP, and supportive therapies. The total number of treatment sessions ranged from 6 to 47. The researchers compared psychotherapy with controls (placebo, TAU, nonspecific control, or waiting list) in eight comparisons and found a mean effect size of $d = 0.23$ (95% CI, 0.06–0.41) in favor of the psychotherapy group, which corresponded with an NNT of 7.69. Heterogeneity was zero ($I^2 = 0$). The effects of psychological treatments were directly compared with those of pharmacotherapy in ten comparisons. The mean effect size was $d = -0.31$ (95% CI, −0.53 to −0.09), which indicated a superior effect of pharmacotherapy ($p < .01$), and which corresponded with an NNT of 5.75. Heterogeneity was moderate to high ($I^2 = 59.03$). In the subgroup analyses, the researchers (Cuijpers, Smit, et al. (2010) found a significant difference between studies in which SSRIs were used, compared with those in which tricyclics were used ($p < .01$), suggesting that SSRIs are more effective than psychotherapy in PDD. In nine comparisons, pharmacotherapy was compared with the combination of pharmacotherapy and psychotherapy. The mean effect size indicating the difference between these two types of treatment was $d = 0.23$ (95% CI, −0.01 to 0.47, $p < .1$) in favor of the combined treatment, which corresponded with an NNT of 7.69. Heterogeneity was moderate ($I^2 = 53.71$).

Further subgroup analyses of this meta-analysis (Cuijpers, Smit, et al. (2010) indicated a significant difference between the effect sizes of studies examining different diagnostic populations, ranging from a negligible effect size for DD patients, to a large effect size for double depression ($p < .01$). The researchers also found a significant difference between SSRIs and other pharmacotherapies (tricyclics or other) ($p < .001$). They also examined four studies in which psychotherapy was compared with the combination of pharmacotherapy and psychotherapy. These four comparisons resulted in an effect size of $d = 0.45$ (95% CI, 0.20–0.70, $p < .001$) in favor of the combined treatment. This corresponds to an NNT of 4.00. Heterogeneity was moderate ($I^2 = 50.90$).

A meta-analysis by Cuijpers et al. (2014) investigated adding psychotherapy to pharmacotherapy in 52 studies of depression and anxiety disorders, with a subset of 32 studies focused only on depressive disorders. The majority of studies ($n = 13$) used CBT, 9 used IPT, and the remaining 10 examined other therapies. The antidepressants that were examined in the studies included SSRIs ($n = 22$), tricyclics ($n = 13$), SNRIs ($n = 3$), monoamine oxidase inhibitors (MAOIs) ($n = 4$), and treatment protocols with different types of antidepressant medication ($n = 10$). The researchers found an overall mean effect size indicating the difference between pharmacotherapy only and combined treatment at posttest for all 52 studies was 0.43 (95% CI, 0.31–0.56) in favor of the combined treatment. This corresponds to an NNT of 4.20, with moderate to high heterogeneity (I^2 = 64, 95% CI, 52–73). The researchers further found that combined treatment was more effective than pharmacotherapy alone in MDD (g = 0.43, 95% CI, 0.29–0.57; NNT = 4.20), and insufficient evidence was found for DD.

Jobst and the European Psychiatric Association Guidance Group (Jobst et al., 2016) also determined that both psychotherapy and pharmacotherapy are effective in PDD, with short-duration psychotherapy found to be less effective when treating DD. They recommended both approaches be used in treating PDD, and proposed a combined evidence level of 1+ (well-conducted meta-analyses, systematic reviews) and grade of A. They advocated that combined treatment is superior to either alone and should be the first treatment approach for chronic MDD but did give the caveat that the evidence does not support any advantage of combined treatment for DD at this time.

Overall, the research appears to support a combined treatment approach as the most effective treatment for PDD. This combined approach would include one of the empirically supported psychotherapies, such as CBASP, IPT, or CBT, and an SSRI, SNRI, NDRI, or tricyclic medication. Research has demonstrated that a combination treatment of pharmacotherapy and psychotherapy extended beyond the initial treatment phase is required for optimal impact on symptom relief and relapse prevention (Hollon et al., 2014; Keller et al., 2000; Thase et al., 1997). It may be helpful to conceptualize PDD as a disorder that must be continuously monitored and one which requires active application of the strategies learned in treatment, much like any other chronic disorder.

> **Research supports a combined treatment approach as the most effective treatment for PDD**

Somatic approaches to treating PDD are typically discussed as options for TRD. TRD is a relative concept, but it is often defined as depression that has not responded to at least two trials of different classes of antidepressants. There is no diagnosis for TRD in the DSM-5. Somatic approaches can be used for TRD and PDD, including ECT, TMS, and VNS. DBS is an emerging approach but lacks extensive research support. ECT remains an important therapeutic option for patients who do not respond to other treatments, and research documents that it is superior to placebo, sham ECT, and antidepressants. The strongest predictor of favorable response to ECT is a history of resistance to antidepressant medications. TMS and VNS are relatively newer somatic treatments, and each has demonstrated effectiveness (Kennedy & Giacobbe, 2007). These somatic treatments may be considered viable options in addition to psychotherapy, especially when antidepressant medications have been unsuccessful.

> **TRD is depression that has not responded to at least 2 trials of different classes of antidepressants**

> **Somatic treatments for PDD include ECT, TMS, and VNS**

4.3 Problems in Carrying Out Treatments

PDD patients may be avoidant, hostile-submissive, and lacking in empathy, insight, and interpersonal skills. They may demonstrate hopeless and helpless behaviors and verbalize unchanging despair, along with an inability to be flexible. All of these characteristics can lead to problems in carrying out effective treatment. It is not surprising, then, that each of the effective psychotherapy approaches for PDD incorporate strategies to help address and overcome these challenges. Issues of noncompliance may interfere with treatment.

> **PDD patients can be challenging as they are often avoidant, passively hostile, hopeless, helpless, and inflexible**

> **Treatment noncompliance is an issue that can interfere with effective treatment**

Noncompliance on the part of a patient may be manifested by hostility toward the therapist, or avoidance behaviors, such as not completing homework.

The PDD patient can discourage and demoralize therapists

IPT provides a framework for therapists to work with discouraging and draining PDD patients. The manualized IPT for dysthymia has contingencies for the therapist to use if an initial IPT strategy has not worked with the patient. The IPT therapist is also encouraged to keep in mind the same message that they are giving to the patient, which is that the patient is not inherently defective but has a treatable disorder. Hopelessness and other avoidance behaviors are conceptualized as some of the treatable symptoms of the PDD patient (Markowitz, 1998).

Advocates of CBT maintain that the first step in addressing noncompliance is to identify and label the problem with the patient (Moore & Garland, 2003). The therapist can then attempt with the patient to understand the avoidance in terms of thoughts or beliefs and to specify predictions from these beliefs that can be tested. The therapy task that is being avoided can then be broken down into smaller steps for the patient to attempt in session with the therapist's support. This is only helpful when the patient attends sessions, and lack of attendance may necessitate more directive approaches on the part of the therapist. Motivational interviewing is conceived of as an adjunct and is indicated for use with clients resistant to and significantly ambivalent about change-based techniques (Westra, 2004).

PDD patients need to be able to engage and respond to therapists

CBASP presents patient skills necessary for the patient to participate effectively: (a) the patient must be able to focus attention on one thing at a time and (b) must be able to shift attention when asked to do so. If these skills are not in place, the therapist can use CPR to clarify the consequences of the patient's behavior in order to shape it. By providing feedback in a safe way to the patient about their interpersonal impact on the therapist, therapy-interfering behaviors can be changed (McCullough, 2000; McCullough 2006; McCullough et al., 2015). An example of how to use CPR is found in Clinical Vignette 2.

Clinical Vignette 2

Use of Contingent Personal Responsivity in CBASP to Facilitate Treatment

Scenario: PDD patient has his head down during initial CBASP sessions and refuses to make eye contact or answer with anything more than one word. This is frustrating for the therapist, and she feels like she is not making any progress. The therapist is tempted to work harder, asking more and more questions.

Instead, the therapist uses contingent personal responsivity (CPR) by pausing and recognizing the interpersonal impact on her: She is being "pulled" into a more dominant and hostile interpersonal stance. With this awareness, the therapist can then reflect on this insight with the patient with the goal of helping the patient understand that he does have an impact on those around him. This is done with great respect and calmness and with the specific learning goal in mind for the patient to understand the impact he is having on the therapist.

The therapist may start by saying something like:

Therapist: I notice that it is hard for you to make eye contact. I wonder if you know how it makes me feel when you do not look at me?
Patient: What? I don't know.
Therapist: Would you like to know how it makes me feel?

Patient: Uh, I guess.
Therapist: OK. It feels very lonely for me.
Patient: Oh, really? I never thought of that....

A conversation has now been initiated, and the therapist can begin to explore the fact that the patient does have some impact on others, and even some control over that impact.

This is an example of a disciplined CPR used with the intent of helping to inform the patient of their stimulus value or interpersonal impact on the therapist.

Psychotherapy for PDD must also be of adequate duration and strength to ensure learning and prevent relapse. Long-term treatment increases the chances of response and remission (Keller, 2002). Most researchers support treatment duration that involves at least 20 weekly sessions with ongoing maintenance therapy sessions indefinitely. Many patients will benefit from a longer duration of treatment (Cuijpers, van Straten, et al., 2010; Jobst et al., 2016), and ongoing maintenance treatment is advised (Keller, 2002; Manber et al., 2008). Many medications for PDD may need to be given at higher doses and for longer periods of time than would be the case for acute or episodic depression (Epstein, Szpindel, & Katzman, 2014).

Psychotherapy and pharmacotherapy must be of adequate duration and strength to facilitate effective treatment

4.4 Multicultural Issues

Clinical trials and research on psychotherapy for PDD within special populations are not abundant. There are no large studies or compelling data regarding psychotherapy effects on PDD in children. One study compared IPT and CBT in Puerto Rican adolescents with MDD; this research found CBT produced statistically significant decreases in depressive symptoms and improved self-concept compared with IPT, with an effect size for CBT versus IPT of 0.43 (Rossello, Bernal, & Rivera-Medina, 2008). No RCTs exploring CBASP for various cultural, ethnic, or age groups have been published, although DeSalvo and McCullough (2002) published a case study of an adolescent female with double depression who was successfully treated with modified CBASP. They reported full remission of the depressive symptoms and acknowledged that modification of the adult form of CBASP was required for successful administration of the therapy. CBT has been adapted for MDD in Hispanics and found to be effective, with statistically significant changes in BDI scores from baseline at posttreatment and at 6-month follow-up (Interian, Allen, Gara, & Escobar, 2008), with an effect size of 2.71. In a study exploring adaptations of CBT for Chinese Americans with severe MDD, Hwang et al. (2015) found that the CBT group displayed a statistically significant decrease in depression (HDRS reduction of 5.53) over 12 sessions ($t = 3.07$, $df=44$, $p = .004$, effect size of $r^2 = .45$) (within-group variance explained), and the culturally adapted-CBT group displayed approximately twice the decrease in depression (HDRS reduction of 10.62) over 12 sessions ($t = 2.16$, $df = 84$, $p = .033$, effect size of $r^2 = .02$). The therapy session effect size was 1.54 and 2.96 for CBT and culturally adapted CBT, respectively.

In a systematic review of depression interventions among racial and ethnic minority older adults over the past 20 years, Fuentes and Aranda (2012) found that favorable depression treatment effects were observed for older minorities across five of the seven studies reviewed. They also found that collaborative or integrated care models were effective specifically with older Latinos and African Americans. They caution, however, that depression treatment effects remain largely unknown for some minority groups, and for distinct racial or ethnic subgroups.

Compliance with treatment, especially pharmacotherapy, may be particularly challenging in certain subpopulations, and researchers have found race and ethnicity to be robust predictors of early antidepressant adherence, with minority groups other than American Indians and Alaska Natives less likely to be adherent (Rossom et al., 2016).

Additional research is needed into multicultural adaptations and applications of psychotherapy for PDD

Supplemental case management has been found to improve retention in CBT administered for depression in ethnic minority groups and may improve outcomes for Spanish-speaking patients with depression (Miranda, Azocar, Organista, Dwyer, & Areane, 2003). Motivational interviewing and culturally sensitive treatment approaches have also been demonstrated to help engage Latino patients with PDD in complying with pharmacotherapy (Interian et al., 2010).

Providing supplemental case management may improve effectiveness and adherence for minorities

The limited work that has been conducted on treatments for PDD in minority populations suggests it is advisable to adapt the treatment as necessary for the population and to also provide additional support or care to help maintain adherence to treatment (Fuentes & Aranda, 2012; Miranda et al., 2003). More research is needed to explore the cultural generalizability of all psychotherapies for PDD and to develop and evaluate cultural adaptations.

Further Reading

For Internet resources, see Appendix 7.

Interpersonal Psychotherapy

Klerman, G. L., Weissman, M. M., Rounsaville, B. J., & Chevron, E. S. (1984). *Interpersonal psychotherapy for depression*. New York, NY: Basic Books.
This is the original IPT manual developed in early IPT studies. It is a textbook that outlines the research and describes the strategies for implementing IPT with depressed patients.

Markowitz, J. C. (1998). *Interpersonal psychotherapy for dysthymic disorder*. Washington, DC: American Psychiatric Press.
This book was developed from the treatment manual used to research IPT for dysthymic disorder. Sections of this book describe in detail the adaptation of IPT for the treatment of dysthymic patients.

Pettit, J. W., & Joiner, T. E. (2005). *The interpersonal solution to depression: A workbook for changing how you feel by changing how you relate*. Oakland, CA: New Harbinger.
This is a workbook describing updated techniques to use in IPT. It can also be used as a self-help book and could be recommended to your depressed patients.

Verdeli, H., & Weissman, M. M. (2019). Interpersonal psychotherapy. In D. Wedding & R. J. Corsini (Eds.), *Current Psychotherapies* (pp. 349–390). Boston, MA: Cengage.
This chapter provides a concise but comprehensive introduction to the current practice of IPT.

Weissman, M. M., Markowitz, J. C., & Klerman, G. L. (2007). *A clinician's guide to interpersonal psychotherapy*. New York, NY: Oxford University Press. http://doi.org/10.1093/med:psych/9780195309416.001.0001
This is a very user-friendly guide for therapist to use to learn and administer IPT. It is meant for clinicians as the name implies and is a good first book to familiarize oneself with IPT.

Cognitive Behavior Therapy

Beck, A. T., Rush, A. J., Shaw, B., & Emery, G. (1979). *Cognitive therapy of depression*. New York, NY: Guilford Press.
This is an early manual on which many of the CBT studies are based. The focus is on depression in general and not persistent depression.

Beck, A. T., & Weishaar, M. (2019). Cognitive therapy. In D. Wedding & R. J. Corsini (Eds.), *Current psychotherapies* (pp. 237–272). Boston, MA: Cengage.
This chapter provides a concise but comprehensive introduction to the current practice of cognitive therapy.

Persons, J. B., Davidson, J., & Tompkins, M. A., (2001). *Essential components of cognitive-behavior therapy for depression*. Washington, DC: American Psychological Association. http://doi.org/10.1037/10389-000
This is a beginner's guide to using CBT with depressed patients, but again the focus is on depression in general and not PDD.

Moore, R. G., & Garland, A. (2003). *Cognitive therapy for chronic and persistent depression.* Chichester, UK: Wiley. http://doi.org/10.1002/9780470713495
This is an excellent manual with details about the research and strategies for using CBT to treat persistent depression. This is the manual used for the Newcastle studies of CBT for chronic depression.

Cognitive Behavioral Analysis System of Psychotherapy

McCullough, J. P., Jr. (2000). *Treatment for chronic depression.* New York, NY: Guilford Press.
This is the original CBASP book that was developed out of the large clinical studies conducted with CBASP. It is an excellent introduction to the basics of CBASP.

McCullough, J. P., Jr. (2001). *Skills training manual for diagnosing and treating chronic depression: cognitive behavioral analysis system of psychotherapy.* New York, NY: Guilford Press.
This is the clinician skills training manual that is meant to accompany the *Treatment for Chronic Depression* book. It is an excellent resource for handouts, and it provides a basic review of CBASP.

McCullough, J. P., Jr. (2002). *Patient's manual for CBASP.* New York, NY: Guilford Press.
This is a manual meant for patients being treated for chronic or persistent depression.

McCullough, J. P., Jr. (2006). *Treating chronic depression with disciplined personal involvement.* New York, NY: Springer.
This is an excellent CBASP book focused on the more challenging components of CBASP therapy – those which involve disciplined interpersonal involvement. The text reviews ethics, as well as strategies including contingent personal responsivity and interpersonal discrimination.

McCullough, J. P., Jr., Schramm, E., & Penberthy, J. K. (2015). *CBASP as a distinctive treatment for persistent depressive disorder.* New York, NY: Routledge.
This is a comprehensive manual for those wishing to learn more about CBASP and how to use it for individuals.

Sayegh, L., & Penberthy, J. K. (2016). *Group treatment manual for persistent depression: Cognitive behavioral analysis system of psychotherapy (CBASP) therapist's guide.* New York, NY: Routledge.
This is a therapist guide for conducting CBASP in a group format. There is also a companion manual for patients published by Routledge. These contain reproducible handouts for patients.

Mindfulness-Based Cognitive Therapy

Williams, J. M. G., Teasdale, J. D., Segal, Z. V., & Kabat-Zinn, J. (2007). *The mindful way through depression: Freeing yourself from chronic unhappiness.* New York, NY: Guilford Press.
This is an introductory book about using mindfulness to prevent relapse in patients who have been treated for depression.

Segal, Z. V., Williams, J. M. G., & Teasdale, J. D. (2013). *Mindfulness-based cognitive therapy for depression* (2nd ed.) New York, NY: Guilford Press.
This is an updated version of the first edition and provides additional research information and materials for delivering MBCT to treat depression as well as prevent relapse.

6

References

aan het Rot, M., Mathew, S. J., & Charney, D. S. (2009). Neurobiological mechanisms in major depressive disorder. *Canadian Medical Association Journal, 180*(3), 305–313. http://doi.org/10.1503/cmaj.080697

Abramson, L. Y., Seligman, M. E., & Teasdale, J. D. (1978). Learned helplessness in humans: Critique and reformulation. *Journal of Abnormal Psychology, 87*(1), 49–74. http://doi.org/10.1037/0021-843X.87.1.49

Abreu, P. R., & Santos, C. E. (2008). Behavioral models of depression: A critique of the emphasis on positive reinforcement. *International Journal of Behavioral Consultation and Therapy, 4*(2), 130–145. http://doi.org/10.1037/h0100838

Agosti, V., & Ocepek-Welikson, K. (1997). The efficacy of imipramine and psychotherapy in early-onset chronic depression: A reanalysis of the National Institute of Mental Health Treatment of Depression Collaborative Research Program. *Journal of Affective Disorders, 43*(3), 181–186.

Akiskal, H., King, D., Rosenthal, T., Robinson, D., & Scott-Strauss, A. (1981). Chronic depressions: Part 1: Clinical and familial characteristics in 137 probands. *Journal of Affective Disorders, 3,* 297–315. http://doi.org/10.1016/0165-0327(81)90031-8

Al-Harbi, K. S. (2012). Treatment-resistant depression: therapeutic trends, challenges, and future directions. *Patient Preference and Adherence, 6,* 369–388. http://doi.org/10.2147/PPA.S29716

American Psychiatric Association. (1994). *Diagnostic and statistical manual of mental disorders* (4th ed.). Washington, DC: Author.

American Psychiatric Association. (2010). *Practice guideline for the treatment of patients with major depressive disorder* (3rd ed.). Washington, DC: Author.

American Psychiatric Association. (2013). *Diagnostic and statistical manual of mental disorders* (5th ed.). Washington, DC: American Psychiatric Publishing. http://doi.org/10.1176/appi.books.9780890425596

Angst, J., Gamma, A., Rossler, W., Ajdacic, V., & Klein, D. (2009). Long-term depression versus episodic major depression: Results from the prospective Zurich study of a community sample. *Journal of Affective Disorders, 115,* 112–121. http://doi.org/10.1016/j.jad.2008.09.023

Bagby, R. M., Ryder, A. G., Schuller, D. R., & Marshall, M. B. (2004). The Hamilton Depression Rating Scale: Has the gold standard become a lead weight? *American Journal of Psychiatry, 161*(12), 2163–2177.

Bair, M. J., Robinson, R. L., Katon, W., & Kroenke, K. (2003). Depression and pain comorbidity: A literature review. *Archives of Internal Medicine, 163*(20), 2433–2445.

Bath, K. G., & Lee, F. S. (2006). Variant BDNF(Val66Met) impact on brain structure and function. *Cognitive, Affective, & Behavioral Neuroscience, 6*(1), 79–85. http://doi.org/10.3758/CABN.6.1.79

Bech, P., Rasmussen, N. A., Olsen, L. R., Noerholm, V., & Abildgaard, W. (2001). The sensitivity and specificity of the Major Depression Inventory, using the Present State Examination as the index of diagnostic validity. *Journal of Affective Disorders, 66*(2-3), 159–164.

Beck, A. T. (1987). Cognitive models of depression. *Journal of Cognitive Psychotherapy: An International Quarterly, 1,* 5–37.

Beck, A. T. (1991). Cognitive therapy a 30-year retrospective. *American Psychologist, 46*(4), 368–375. http://doi.org/10.1037/0003-066X.46.4.368

Beck, A. T., Rush, A. J., Shaw, B. F., & Emery, G. (1979). *Cognitive therapy of depression.* New York, NY: Guilford.

Beck, A. T., Steer, R. A., & Brown, G. K. (1996). *Manual for the Beck Depression Inventory–II.* San Antonio, TX: Psychological Corporation.

Beck, A. T., Weissman, A., Lester, D., & Trexler, L. (1974). The measurement of pessimism: The hopelessness scale. *Journal of Consulting and Clinical Psychology, 42*(6), 861–865. http://doi.org/10.1037/h0037562

Beck, J. S. (2011). *Cognitive behavior therapy: Basics and beyond* (2nd ed.). New York, NY: Guilford Press.

Beckham, E. E. (1990). Psychotherapy of depression at the crossroads: Directions for the 1990s. *Clinical Psychology Review, 10,* 207–228. http://doi.org/10.1016/0272-7358(90)90058-I

Blanco, C., Okuda, M., Markowitz, J. C., Liu, S. M., Grant, B. F., & Hasin, D. S. (2010). The epidemiology of chronic major depressive disorder and dysthymic disorder: Results from the National Epidemiologic Survey on Alcohol and Related Conditions. *The Journal of Clinical Psychiatry, 71*(12), 1645–1656.

Bradley, R. G., Binder, E. B., Epstein, M. P., Tang, Y., Nair, H. P., Liu, W., … Gold, P. W. (2008). Influence of child abuse on adult depression: Moderation by the corticotropin-releasing hormone receptor gene. *Archives of General Psychiatry, 65*(2), 190–200. http://doi.org/10.1001/archgenpsychiatry.2007.26

Brown, G., Craig, T. K., & Harris, T. O. (2008). Parental maltreatment and proximal risk factors using the Childhood Experiences of Care & Abuse (CECA) instrument: A life-course study of adult chronic depression. *Journal of Affective Disorders, 110,* 222–233. http://doi.org/10.1016/j.jad.2008.01.016

Budge, S. L., Adelson, J. L., & Howard, K. A. (2013). Anxiety and depression in transgender individuals: The roles of transition status, loss, social support, and coping. *Journal of Consulting and Clinical Psychology, 81*(3), 545–557. http://doi.org/10.1037/a0031774

Byers, A. L., Yaffe, K., Covinsky, K. E., Friedman, M. B., & Bruce, M. L. (2010). High occurrence of mood and anxiety disorders among older adults: The national comorbidity survey replication. *Archives of General Psychiatry, 67*(5), 489–496. http://doi.org/10.1001/archgenpsychiatry.2010.35

Carter, J. D., McIntosh, V. V., Jordan, J., Porter, R. J., Frampton, C. M., & Joyce, P. R. (2013). Psychotherapy for depression: A randomized clinical trial comparing schema therapy and cognitive behavior therapy. *Journal of Affective Disorders, 151,* 500–505. http://doi.org/10.1016/j.jad.2013.06.034

Carver, C. S., Scheier, M., & Weintraub, J. K. (1989). Assessing coping strategies: A theoretically based approach. *Journal of Personality and Social Psychology, 56,* 267–283. http://doi.org/10.1037/0022-3514.56.2.267

Caspi, A., Sugden, K., Moffitt, T. E., Taylor, A., Craig, J. W., Harrington, H., … Poulton, R. (2003). Influence of life stress on depression: Moderation by a polymorphism in the 5-HTT gene. *Science, 301*(5631), 386–389.

Chambers, W. J., Puig-Antich, J., Hirsch, M., Paez, P., Ambrosini, P. J., Tabrizi, M. A., Davies, M. (1985). The assessment of affective disorders in children and adolescents by semistructured interview. Test-retest reliability of the schedule for affective disorders and schizophrenia for school-age children, present episode version. *Archives of General Psychiatry, 42*(7), 696–702.

Clements-Nolle, K., Marx, R., Guzman, R., & Katz, M. (2001). HIV prevalence, risk behaviors, health care use, and mental health status of transgender persons: Implications for public health intervention. *American Journal of Public Health, 91*(6), 915–921. http://doi.org/10.2105/AJPH.91.6.915

Cohen, S., Kamarck, T., & Mermelstein, R. (1983). A global measure of perceived stress. *Journal of Health and Social Behavior, 24,* 385–396. http://doi.org/10.2307/2136404

Constantino, M. J., Manber, R., Degeorge, J., McBride, C., Ravitz, P., Zuroff, D. C., … Arnow, B. A. (2008). Interpersonal styles of chronically depressed outpatients: Profiles and therapeutic change. *Psychotherapy, 45*(4), 491–506. http://doi.org/10.1037/a0014335

Cools, R., Calder, A. J., Lawrence, A. D., Clark, L., Bullmore, E., & Robbins, T. W. (2005). Individual differences in threat sensitivity predict serotonergic modulation of amygdala response to fearful faces. *Psychopharmacology, 189*(4), 670–679. http://doi.org/10.1007/s00213-005-2215-5

Cuijpers, P., Geraedts, A. S., van Oppen, P., Andersson, G., Markowitz, J. C., & van Straten, A. (2011). Interpersonal psychotherapy for depression: A meta-analysis. *American Journal of Psychiatry, 168*(6), 581–952. http://doi.org/10.1176/appi.ajp.2010.10101411

Cuijpers, P., Reynolds, C. F., Donker, T., Li, J., Andersson, G., & Beekman, A. (2012). Personalized treatment of adult depression: Medication, psychotherapy, or both? A systematic review. *Depression and Anxiety, 29,* 855–864. http://doi.org/10.1002/da.21985

Cuijpers, P., Sijbrandij, M., Koole, S. L., Andersson, G., Beekman, A. T., & Reynolds, C. F. (2014). Adding psychotherapy to antidepressant medication in depression and anxiety disorders: A meta-analysis. *World Psychiatry, 13*(1), 56–67. http://doi.org/10.1002/wps.20089

Cuijpers, P., Smit, F., Bohlmeijer, E., Hollon, S. D., & Andersson, G. (2010). Efficacy of cognitive-behavioural therapy and other psychological treatments for adult depression: Meta-analytic study of publication bias. *British Journal of Psychiatry, 196*(3), 173–178.

Cuijpers, P., van Straten, A., Schuurmans, J., van Oppen, P., Hollon, S. D., & Andersson, G. (2010). Psychotherapy for chronic major depression and dysthymia: A meta-analysis. *Clinical Psychology Review, 30*(1), 51–62. http://doi.org/10.1016/j.cpr.2009.09.003

Cuijpers, P., van Straten, A., Warmerdam, L., & Andersson, G. (2009). Psychotherapy versus the combination of psychotherapy and pharmacotherapy in the treatment of depression: A meta-analysis. *Depression and Anxiety, 26*(3), 279–288. http://doi.org/10.1002/da.20519

Derogatis, L. R. (1993). *The Brief Symptom Inventory (BSI): Administration, scoring and procedures manual.* Minneapolis, MN: National Computer Systems.

DeRubeis, R. J., Gelfand, L. A., Tang, T. Z., & Simons, A. D. (1999). Medications versus cognitive behavior therapy for severely depressed outpatients: Mega-analysis of four randomized comparisons. *American Journal of Psychiatry, 156*(7), 1007–1013.

Dhejne, C., Lichtenstein, P., Bowman, M., Johannson, A. L., Långström, N., & Landén, M. (2011). Long-term follow-up of transsexual persons undergoing sex reassignment surgery: Cohort study in Sweden. *PLoS ONE , 6*(2), e16885. http://doi.org/10.1371/journal.pone.0016885

Djernes, J. K. (2006). Prevalence and predictors of depression in populations of elderly: A review. *Acta Psychiatry Scandanavia, 113*(5), 372–87. http://doi.org/10.1111/j.1600-0447.2006.00770.x

Dolnak, D. R. (2006). Treating patients for comorbid depression, anxiety disorders, and somatic illnesses. *Journal of the American Osteopathic Association, 106*(S2), 1S-8S.

Donker, T., Griffiths, K. M., Cuijpers, P., & Christensen, H. (2009). Psychoeducation for depression, anxiety and psychological distress: A meta-analysis. *BMC Medicine, 7*(79), 1–9. http://doi.org/10.1186/1741-7015-7-79

Ellis, A., & Grieger, R. (1977). *RET: Handbook of rational-emotive therapy.* New York, NY: Springer.

Elovainio, M., Jokela, M., Kivimaki, M., Pulkki-Raback, L., Lehtimaki, T., Airla, N., … Keltikangas-Jarvinen, L. (2007). Genetic variants in the DRD2 gene moderate the relationship between stressful life events and depressive symptoms in adults: Cardiovascular risk in young Finns study. *Psychosomatic Medicine, 69*(5), 391–395.

Epstein, I., Szpindel, I., & Katzman, M. A. (2014). Pharmacological approaches to manage persistent symptoms of major depressive disorder: Rationale and therapeutic strategies. *Psychiatry Research, 220*(S1), S15–S33. http://doi.org/10.1016/S0165-1781(14)70003-4

Fava, G. A., Rafanelli, C., Grandi, S., Conti, S., & Belluardo, P. (1998). Prevention of recurrent depression with cognitive behavioral therapy: Preliminary findings. *Archives of General Psychiatry, 55*(9), 816–820. http://doi.org/10.1001/archpsyc.55.9.816

Ferster, C. H. (1973). A functional analysis of depression. *American Psychologist, 28,* 857–870.

First, M. B., Williams, J. B. W., Karg, R. S., Spitzer, R. L. (2015). Structured Clinical Interview for DSM-5 – Research Version (SCID-5 for DSM-5, Research Version; SCID-5-RV). Arlington, VA: American Psychiatric Association.

Flanagan, J. C. (1982). Measurement of quality of life: Current state of the art. *Archives of Physical Medicine and Rehabilitation, 63*(2), 56–59.

Folkman, S., & Lazarus, R. S. (1988). Coping as a mediator of emotion. *Journal of Personality and Social Psychology, 54*(3), 466–475. http://doi.org/10.1037/0022-3514.54.3.466

Fournier, J. C., DeRubeis, R. J., Hollon, S. D., Dimidjian, S., Amsterdam, J. D., Shelton, R. C., et al. (2010). Antidepressant drug effects and depression severity: A patient-level meta-analysis. *Journal of the American Medical Association, 303*(1), 47–53. http://doi.org/10.1001/jama.2009.1943

Fuchs, C. Z., & Rehm, L. P. (1977). A self-control behavior therapy program for depression. *Journal of Consulting and Clinical Psychology, 45*(2), 206–215. http://doi.org/10.1037/0022-006X.45.2.206

Fuentes, D., & Aranda, M. P. (2012). Depression interventions among racial and ethnic minority older adults: A systematic review across 20 years. *American Journal of Geriatric Psychiatry, 20*(11), 915–931. http://doi.org/10.1097/JGP.0b013e31825d091a

Garyfallos, G., Adarnopoulou, A., Karastergiou, A., Voikli, K., Sotiropoulou, A., Donias, S.,… Paraschos, A.. (1999). Personality disorders in dysthymia and major depression. *Acta Psychiatrica Scandinavica, 99*(5), 332–340. http://doi.org/10.1111/j.1600-0447.1999.tb07238.x

Gelenberg, A. J., Kocsis, J. H., McCullough, J. P., Ninan, P. T., & Thase, M. E. (2006). The state of knowledge of chronic depression. *Primary Care Companion to the Journal of Clinical Psychiatry, 8*(2), 60–65. http://doi.org/10.4088/PCC.v08n0201

Gloaguen, V., Cottraux, J., Cucherat, M., Blackburn, I. (1998). A meta-analysis of the effects of cognitive therapy in depressed patients. *Journal of Affective Disorders, 49,* 59–72. http://doi.org/10.1016/S0165-0327(97)00199-7

Goethe, J. W., Fischer, E. H., & Wright, J. S. (1993). Severity as a key construct in depression. *Journal of Nervous and Mental Disorders, 181*(12), 718–724. http://doi.org/10.1097/00005053-199312000-00002

Goodwin, G. M. (2006). Depression and associated physical disease and symptoms. *Dialogues in Clinical Neuroscience, 8*(2), 259–265.

Grant, B. F., Stinson, F. S., Dawson, D. A., Chou, S. P., Dufour, M. C., Compton, W., … Kaplan, K. (2004). Prevalence and co-occurrence of substance use disorders and independent mood and anxiety disorders: Results from the National Epidemiologic Survey on Alcohol and Related Conditions. *Archives of General Psychiatry, 61*(8), 807–816.

Griffiths, J., Ravindran, A. V., Merali, Z., & Anisman, H. (2000). Dysthymia: A review of pharmacological and behavioral factors. *Molecular Psychiatry, 5*(3), 242–261. http://doi.org/10.1038/sj.mp.4000697

Gu, J., Strauss, C., Bond, R., & Cavanagh, K. (2015). How do mindfulness-based cognitive therapy and mindfulness-based stress reduction improve mental health and wellbeing? A systematic review and meta-analysis of mediation studies. *Clinical Psychology Review, 37,* 1–12.

Hajek, T., Kozeny, J., Kopecek, M., Alda, M., & Höschl, C. (2008). Reduced subgenual cingulate volumes in mood disorders: A meta-analysis. *Journal of Psychiatry and Neuroscience, 33*(2), 91–99.

Hames, J. L., Hagan, C. R., & Joiner, T. E. (2013). Interpersonal processes in depression. *Annual Review of Clinical Psychology, 9,* 355–377. http://doi.org/10.1146/annurev-clinpsy-050212-185553

Hamilton, M. (1960). A rating scale for depression. *Journal of Neurology, Neurosurgery, and Psychiatry, 23,* 56–62. http://doi.org/10.1136/jnnp.23.1.56

Hammen, C., Brennan, P. A., Keenan-Miller, D., Herr, N. R. (2008). Early onset recurrent subtype of adolescent depression: Clinical and psychosocial correlates. *Journal of Child Psychology and Psychiatry, 49,* 433–440. http://doi.org/10.1111/j.1469-7610.2007.01850.x

Hardeveld, F., Spijker, J., De Graaf, R., Hendriks, S. M., Licht, C. M., Nolen, W. A., … Beekman, A. T. (2013). Recurrence of major depressive disorder across different treatment settings: Results from the NESDA study. *Journal of Affective Disorders, 147*(1-3), 225–231.

Hashimoto, K. (2009). Emerging role of glutamate in the pathophysiology of major depressive disorder. *Brain Research Reviews, 61*(2), 105–123. http://doi.org/10.1016/j.brainresrev.2009.05.005

Hasin, D. S., Goodwin, R. D., Stinson, F. S., & Grant, B. F. (2005). Epidemiology of major depressive disorder: Results from the National Epidemiologic Survey on Alcoholism and Related Conditions. *Archives of General Psychiatry, 62*(10), 1097–1106. http://doi.org/10.1001/archpsyc.62.10.1097

Heim, C., & Binder, E. B. (2012). Current research trends in early life stress and depression: Review of human studies on sensitive periods, gene-environment interactions, and epigenetics. *Experimental Neurology, 233*(1), 102–111. http://doi.org/10.1016/j.expneurol.2011.10.032

Heim, C., Bradley, B., Mletzko, T. C., Deveau, T. C., Musselman, D. L., Nemeroff, C. B., … Binder, E. B. (2009). Effect of childhood trauma on adult depression and neuroendocrine function: Sex-specific moderation by CRH Receptor 1 Gene. *Frontiers of Behavioral Neuroscience, 3*, 41.

Hendrie, H. C., Albert, M. S., Butters, M. A., Gao, S., Knopman, D. S., Launer, L. J., … Wagster, M. V. (2006). The NIH Cognitive and Emotional Health Project. Report of the Critical Evaluation Study Committee. *Alzheimers and Dementia, 2*(1), 12–32. http://doi.org/10.1016/j.jalz.2005.11.004

Hoffman, S. G., Asnaani, A., Vonk, J., Sawyer, A. T., & Fang, A. (2012). The efficacy of cognitive behavioral therapy: A review of meta-analyses. *Cognitive Therapy Research, 36*(5), 427–440. http://doi.org/10.1007/s10608-012-9476-1

Hollon, S. D., DeRubeis, R. J., Fawcett, J., Amsterdam, J. D., Shelton, R. C., Zajecka, J., … Gallop, R. (2016). Notice of retraction and replacement. *Journal of the American Medical Association Psychiatry, 73*(6), 639–640.

Hollon, S. D., & Kendall, P. C. (1980). Cognitive self-statements in depression: Development of an automatic thoughts questionnaire. *Cognitive Therapy and Research, 4,* 383–395. http://doi.org/10.1007/BF01178214

Hollon, S. D., DeRubeis, R. J., Fawcett, J., Amsterdam, J. D., Shelton, R. C., Zajecka, J., Young, P. R., & Gallop, R. (2014). Effect of cognitive therapy with antidepressant medications vs antidepressants alone on the rate of recovery in major depressive disorder: A randomized clinical trial. *JAMA Psychiatry, 71*(10), 1157–1164.

Howland, R. H., & Thase, M. E. (1991). Biological studies of dysthymia. *Biological Psychiatry, 30*(3), 283–304. http://doi.org/10.1016/0006-3223(91)90112-Y

Hwang, W. C., Meyers, H., Chiu, E., Mak, E., Butner, J., Fujimoto, K., … Miranda, J. (2015). Culturally adapted cognitive behavioral therapy for depressed Chinese Americans: A randomized controlled trial. *Psychiatric Services, 66*(10), 1035–1042. http://doi.org/10.1176/appi.ps.201400358

Ingram, R. E., Miranda, J., & Segal, Z. V. (1998). *Cognitive vulnerability to depression.* New York, NY: Guilford Press.

Interian, A., Allen, L. A., Gara, M. A., & Escobar, J. I. (2008). A pilot study of culturally adapted cognitive behavior therapy for Hispanics with major depression. *Cognitive and Behavioral Practice, 15,* 67–75. http://doi.org/10.1016/j.cbpra.2006.12.002

Interian, A., Ang, A., Gara, M. A., Link, B. G., Rodriguez, M. A., & Vega, W. A. (2010). Stigma and depression treatment utilization among Latinos: Utility of four stigma measures. *Psychiatric Services, 61*(4), 373–379. http://doi.org/10.1176/ps.2010.61.4.373

Jacobson, N. S., Martell, C. R., & Dimidjian, S. (2001). Behavioral activation for depression: Returning to contextual roots. *Clinical Psychology: Science and Practice, 8,* 255–270. http://doi.org/10.1093/clipsy.8.3.255

Jans, L. A., Riedel, W. J., Markus, C. R., & Blokland, A. (2007). Serotonergic vulnerability and depression: Assumptions, experimental evidence and implications. *Molecular Psychiatry, 12,* 522–543. http://doi.org/10.1038/sj.mp.4001920

Jarrett, R. B., Kraft, D., Doyle, J., Foster, B. M., Eaves, G. G., & Silver, P. C. (2001). Preventing recurrent depression using cognitive therapy with and without a continuation phase: A randomized clinical trial. *Archives of General Psychiatry, 58,* 381–388.

Jobst, A., Brakemeier, E. L., Buchheim, A., Caspar, F., Cuijpers, P., Ebmeier, K. P., … Padberg, F. (2016). European Psychiatric Association guidance on psychotherapy in chronic depression across Europe. *European Psychiatry, 33,* 18–36. http://doi.org/10.1016/j.eurpsy.2015.12.003

Kang, H. J., Kim, S. Y., Bae, K. Y., Kim, S. W., Shin, I. S., Yoon, J. S., … Kim, J. M. (2015). Comorbidity of depression with physical disorders: Research and clinical implications. *Chonnam Medical Journal, 51*(1), 8–18. http://doi.org/10.4068/cmj.2015.51.1.8

Katon, W. J. (2011). Epidemiology and treatment of depression in patients with chronic medical illness. *Dialogues in Clinical Neuroscience, 13*(1), 7–23.

Keller, M. B. (1990). Diagnostic and course of Illness variables pertinent to refractory depression. In S. M. A. Tasman (Ed.), *Review of Psychiatry* (Vol. 9, pp. 10–32). Washington, DC: American Psychiatric Press.

Keller, M. B. (2002). Rationale and options for the long-term treatment of depression. *Human Psychopharmacology, 17*(S1), S43–S46. http://doi.org/10.1002/hup.400

Keller, M. (2013). Major depressive disorder: Long-Term course, treatment, and complications. *Psychiatric News, 48*(18), 1–1. http://doi.org/10.1176/appi.pn.2013.9b23

Keller, M. B., Klein, D. N., Hirschfeld, R. M. A., Kocsis, J. H., McCullough, J. P., Jr., Miller, I., First, M. B., Holzer, C. P., III., Keitner, G. I., Marin, D. B., & Shea, T. (1995). Results of the DSM-IV Mood Disorders Field Trial. *American Journal of Psychiatry, 152,* 843–849.

Keller, M. B., McCullough, J. P., Klein, D. N., Arnow, B., Dunner, D. L., Gelenberg, A. J., … Zajecka, J. (2000). A comparison of nefazodone, the cognitive behavioral-analysis system of psychotherapy, and their combination for the treatment of chronic depression. *New England Journal of Medicine, 342,* 1462–1470.

Kendler, K. S., Gardner, C. O., & Prescott, C. A. (2002). Toward a comprehensive developmental model for major depression in women. *American Journal of Psychiatry, 159,* 1133–1145. http://doi.org/10.1176/appi.ajp.159.7.1133

Kennedy, S. H., & Giacobbe, P. (2007). Treatment resistant depression: Advances in somatic therapies. *Annals of Clinical Psychiatry, 19*(4), 279–287. http://doi.org/10.1080/10401230701675222

Kessler, R. C., Berglund, P., Demler, O., Jin, R., Koretz, D., & Merikangas, K. R. (2003). The epidemiology of major depressive disorder: Results from the National Comorbidity Survey Replication (NCS-R). *Journal of the American Medical Association, 289*(23), 3095–3105. http://doi.org/10.1001/jama.289.23.3095

Kessler, R. C., Berglund, P., Demler, O., Jin, R., Merikangas, K. R., & Walters, E. E. (2005). Lifetime prevalence and age-of-onset distributions of DSM-IV disorders in the National Comorbidity Survey Replication. *Archives of General Psychiatry, 62*(6), 593–602. http://doi.org/10.1001/archpsyc.62.6.593

Kessler, R. C., & Bromet, E. J. (2013). The epidemiology of depression across cultures. *Annual Review of Public Health, 34,* 119–138. http://doi.org/10.1146/annurev-publhealth-031912-114409

Kiesler, D. J., & Schmidt, J. A. (2006). *The Impact Message Inventory – Circumplex (IMI-C).* Menlo Park, CA: Mind Garden.

Kim, J. S., Schmid-Burgk, W., Claus, D., & Kornhuber, H. H. (1982). Increased serum glutamate in depressed patients. *Archiv für Psychiatrie und Nervenkrankheiten, 232*(4), 299–304. http://doi.org/10.1007/BF00345492

Klein, D. N., Leon, A. C., D'Zurilla, T. J., Black, S. R., Vivian, D., Dowling, F., … Kocsis, J. H. (2011). Social problem solving and depressive symptoms over time: A randomized clinical trial of cognitive-behavioral analysis system of psychotherapy, brief supportive psychotherapy, and pharmacotherapy. *Journal of Consulting and Clinical Psychology, 79*(3), 342–352.

Klein, D. N., & Santiago, N. J. (2003). Dysthymia and chronic depression: Introduction, classification, risk factors, and course. *Journal of Clinical Psychology, 59,* 807–816. http://doi.org/10.1002/jclp.10174

Klein, D. N., Santiago, N. J., Vivian, D., Blalock, J. A., Kocsis, J. H., Markowitz, J. C., … Keller, M. B. (2004). Cognitive-behavioral analysis system of psychotherapy as a maintenance treatment for chronic depression. *Journal of Consulting and Clinical Psychology, 72*(4), 681–688.

Klein, D. N., Schatzberg, A. F., McCullough, J. P., Keller, M. B., Dowling, F., Goodman, D., … Harrison, W. D. (1999). Early- versus late-onset dysthymic disorder: Comparison in outpatients with superimposed major depressive episodes. *Journal of Affective Disorder, 52,* 187–196.

Klein, D. N., Shankman, S. A., & Rose, S. (2008). Dysthymic disorder and double depression: Prediction of 10-year course trajectories and outcomes. *Journal of Psychiatric Research, 42*(5), 408–415. http://doi.org/10.1016/j.jpsychires.2007.01.009

Klein, J. P., Roniger, A., Schweiger, U., Späth, C., & Brodbeck, J. (2015). The association of childhood trauma and personality disorders with chronic depression: A cross-sectional study in depressed outpatients. *Journal of Clinical Psychiatry, 76*(6), 794–801. http://doi.org/10.4088/JCP.14m09158

Klerman, G. L., Weissman, M. M., Rounsaville, B. J., & Chevron, E. (1984). *Interpersonal psychotherapy of depression.* New York, NY: Basic Books.

Kocsis, J. H., Gelenberg, A., Rothbaum, B. O., Klein, D. N., Trivedi, M. H., Manber, R., … REVAMP Investigators. (2009). Cognitive behavioral analysis system of psychotherapy and brief supportive psychotherapy for augmentation of antidepressant nonresponse in chronic depression: The REVAMP Trial. *Archives of General Psychiatry, 66*(11), 1178–1188.

Kornstein, S. G., & Schneider, R. K. (2001). Clinical features of treatment-resistant depression. *Journal of Clinical Psychiatry, 62*(Suppl 16), 18–25.

Kounou, K. B., Bui, E., Dassa, K. S., Hinton, D., Fischer, L., Djassoa, G., … Schmitt, L. (2013). Childhood trauma, personality disorders symptoms and current major depressive disorder in Togo. *Social Psychiatry and Psychiatric Epidemiology, 48*(7), 1095–1103. http://doi.org/10.1007/s00127-012-0634-2

Kriston, L., von Wolff, A., Westphal, A., Hölzel, L. P., & Härter, M. (2014). Efficacy and acceptability of acute treatments for persistent depressive disorder: a network meta-analysis. *Depression and Anxiety, 31*(8), 621–630. http://doi.org/10.1002/da.22236

Kroenke, K., Spitzer, R. L., & Williams, J. B. (2001). The PHQ-9 validity of a Brief Depression Severity Measure. *Journal of General Internal Medicine, 16*(9), 606–613. http://doi.org/10.1046/j.1525-1497.2001.016009606.x

Kuehner, C. (1999). Gender differences in the short-term course of unipolar depression in a follow-up sample of depressed inpatients. *Journal of Affective Disorders, 56*(2-3), 127–39. http://doi.org/10.1016/S0165-0327(99)00035-X

Kuyken, W., Hayes, R., Barrett, B., Byng, R., Dalgleish, T., Kessler, D., … Byford, S. (2015). Effectiveness and cost-effectiveness of mindfulness-based cognitive therapy compared with maintenance antidepressant treatment in the prevention of depressive relapse or recurrence (PREVENT): A randomised controlled trial. *Lancet, 386*(9988), 63–73.

Lee, H. B. (1990). Reliability, validity and fakability of the Zung self-rating Depression Scale. *Bulletin of the Hong Kong Psychological Society*, 24–25, 5–15.

Lewinsohn, P. M., & Talkington, J. (1979). Studies on the measurement of unpleasant events and relations with depression. *Applied Psychological Measurement, 3*(1), 83–101.

Lewinsohn, P. M., Hoberman, H. M., Teri, L., & Hautzinger, M. (1985). An integrative theory of depression. In S. R. Bootzin (Ed.), *Theoretical issues in behavior therapy* (pp. 331–359). Orlando, FL: Academic Press.

Lewinsohn, P. M., Hops, H., Roberts, R. E., Seeley, J. R., & Andrews, J. A. (1993). Adolescent psychopathology: Part I: Prevalence and incidence of depression and other DSM-III-R disorders in high school students. *Journal of Abnormal Psychology, 102*(1), 133–44. http://doi.org/10.1037/0021-843X.102.1.133

Lewinsohn, P., Mischel, W., Chaplin, W., & Barton, R. (1980). Social competence and depression: The role of illusory self-perception. *Journal of Abnormal Psychology, 89,* 203–212. http://doi.org/10.1037/0021-843X.89.2.203

Lewinsohn, P. M., & Talkington, J. (1979). Studies on the measurement of unpleasant events and relations with depression. *Applied Psychological Measurement, 3*(1), 83–101. http://doi.org/10.1177/014662167900300110

Ley, P. S., Helbig-Lang, S., Czilwik, S., Lang, T., Worlitz, A., Brucher, K., … Petermann, F. (2011). Phenomenological differences between acute and chronic forms of depression in inpatients. *Nordic Journal of Psychiatry, 65*, 330–337.

Linde, K., Kriston, L., Rucker, G., Jamil, S., Schumann, I., Meissner, K., … Schneider, A. (2015). Efficacy and acceptability of pharmacological treatments for depressive disorders in primary care: Systematic review and network meta-analysis. *Annals of Family Medicine, 13*(1), 69–79.

Lobbestael, J., Leurgans, M., & Arntz, A. (2011). Inter-rater reliability of the Structured Clinical Interview for DSM-IV Axis I Disorders (SCID I) and Axis II Disorders (SCID II). *Clinical Psychology & Psychotherapy, 18*(1), 75–79. http://doi.org/10.1002/cpp.693

Locke, K. D., Sayegh, L., Penberthy, J. K., Weber, C., Haentjens, K., & Turecki, G. (2017). Interpersonal circumplex profiles of persistent depression: Goals, self-efficacy, problems, and effects of group therapy. *Journal of Clinical Psychology, 73*(6), 595–611. http://doi.org/10.1002/jclp.22343

Locke, K. D., Sayegh, L., Weber, C., & Turecki, G. (2016). Interpersonal self-efficacy, goals, and problems of persistently depressed outpatients: Prototypical circumplex profiles and distinctive subgroups. *Assessment, 25*(8), 988–1000.

Lohoff, F. W. (2010). Overview of the genetics of major depressive disorder. *Current Psychiatric Reports, 12*(6), 539–546. http://doi.org/10.1007/s11920-010-0150-6

Lucassen, M. F., Stasiak, K., Samra, R., Frampton, C. M., & Merry, S. N. (2017). Sexual minority youth and depressive symptoms or depressive disorder: A systematic review and meta-analysis of population-based studies. *Australian and New Zealand Journal of Psychiatry, 51*(8), 774–787.

Lyketsos, C. G., Nestadt, G., Cwi, J., Heithof, K., & Eaton, W. W. (1994). The life-chart method to describe the course of psychopathology. *International Journal of Methods in Psychiatric Research, 4,* 143–155.

MacKenzie, M. B., & Kocovski, N. L. (2016). Mindfulness-based cognitive therapy for depression: Trends and developments. *Psychology Research and Behavior Management, 9,* 125–132.

MacPhillamy, D. J., & Lewinsohn, P. M. (1982). The pleasant events schedule: Studies on reliability, validity, and scale intercorrelation. *Journal of Consulting and Clinical Psychology, 50*(3), 363–380. http://doi.org/10.1037/0022-006X.50.3.363

Main, M., Goldwyn, R., & Hesse, E. (2002). *Adult attachment scoring and classification system.* Unpublished manuscript, University of California at Berkeley, Berkeley, CA, USA.

Manber, R., Kraemer, H. C., Arnow, B. A., Trivedi, M. H., Rush, A. J., Thase, M. E., … Keller, M. E. (2008). Faster remission of chronic depression with combined psychotherapy and medication than with each therapy alone. *Journal of Consulting and Clinical Psychology, 76*(3), 459–467.

Markowitz, J. C. (1998). *Interpersonal psychotherapy for dysthymic disorder.* Washington, DC: American Psychiatric Publishing.

Markowitz, J. C. (2003). Interpersonal psychotherapy for chronic depression. *Journal of Clinical Psychology, 59,* 847–858. http://doi.org/10.1002/jclp.10177

Markowitz, J. C., Bleiberg, K. L., Christos, P., & Levitan, E. (2006). Solving interpersonal problems correlates with symptom improvement in interpersonal psychotherapy: Preliminary findings. *Journal of Nervous and Mental Disorders, 194*(1), 15–20. http://doi.org/10.1097/01.nmd.0000195314.80210.41

Markowitz, J. C., Leon, A. C., Miller, N. L., & Villalobos, L. (2000). Rater agreement on interpersonal psychotherapy problem areas. *Journal of Psychotherapy Practice and Research, 9*(3), 131–135.

Markowitz, J. C., & Weissman, M. M. (2004). Interpersonal psychotherapy: Principles and applications. *World Psychiatry, 3*(3), 136–139.

Martell, C. R., Addis, M. E., & Jacobson, N. S. (2001). *Depression in context: Strategies for guided action.* New York, NY: W. W. Norton.

Martinowich, K., Manji, H., & Lu, B. (2007). New insights into BDNF function in depression and anxiety. *Nature Neuroscience, 10*(9), 1089–1093. http://doi.org/10.1038/nn1971

McClung, C. A., & Nestler, E. J. (2008). Neuroplasticity mediated by altered gene expression. *Neuropsychopharmacology, 33*(1), 3–17. http://doi.org/10.1038/sj.npp.1301544

McCullough, J. P., Jr. (2000). *Treatment for chronic depression: Cognitive behavioral analysis system of psychotherapy (CBASP)*. New York, NY: Guilford Press.

McCullough, J. P., Jr. (2002). *Patient's manual for CBASP*. New York, NY: Guilford Press.

McCullough, J. P., Jr. (2003). *Patient's manual for CBASP*. New York, NY: Guilford Press.

McCullough, J. P. (2006). *Treating chronic depression with disciplined personal involvement*. New York, NY: Springer.

McCullough, J. P., Jr. (2012a). Introduction and state-of-the-art issues for CBASP. In F. C. M. Belz (Ed.), *CBASP in practice: Basic concepts and new developments*. Munich, Germany: Elsevier.

McCullough, J. P., Jr. (2012b). The way early-onset chronically depressed patients are treated today makes me sad. *Open Journal of Psychiatry, 2,* 9–11.

McCullough, J. P., Jr. (2018). *CBASP training workbook*. Unpublished training manuscript.

McCullough, J. P., Jr. Braith, J. A., Chapman, R. C., Kasnetz, M. D., Carr, K. F., Cones, J. H., … Roberts, W. C. (1990). Comparison of early and late-onset dysthymia. *Journal of Nervous and Mental Diseases, 176,* 658–667. http://doi.org/10.1097/00005053-199009000-00004

McCullough, J. P., Jr., Clark, S. W., Klein, D. N., & First, M. B. (2016a). A procedure to graph the quality of psychosocial functioning affected by symptom severity. *American Journal of Psychotherapy, 70*(2), 222–231.

McCullough, J. P., Jr., Clark, S. W., Klein, D. N., & First, M. B. (2016b). Introducing a clinical course-graphing scale for DSM-5 mood disorders. *American Journal of Psychotherapy, 70*(4), 383–392.

McCullough, J. P., Jr., Kornstein, S. G., McCullough, J. P., Belyea-Caldwell, S., Kaye, A. L., Roberts, W. C., … Kruus, L. (1996). Differential diagnosis of the chronic depressions. *Psychiatric Clinics of North America, 19,* 55–71. http://doi.org/10.1016/S0193-953X(05)70273-2

McCullough, J. P., Jr., Schramm, E., & Penberthy, J. K. (2015). *CBASP: A distinctive treatment for persistent depressive disorder*. New York, NY: Routledge.

McDowell, I. (2006). *Measuring health: A guide to rating scales and questionnaires* (3rd ed.). New York, NY: Oxford Press. http://doi.org/10.1093/acprof:oso/9780195165678.001.0001

Merikangas, K. R., He, J., Burstein, M., Swanson, S. A., Avenevoli, S., Cui, L., … Swendsen, J. (2010). Lifetime prevalence of mental disorders in US adolescents: Results from the National Comorbidity Study-Adolescent Supplement (NCS-A). *Journal of American Academy of Child and Adolescent Psychiatry, 49*(10), 980–989.

Merikangas, K. R., & Swendsen, J. D. (1997). Genetic epidemiology of psychiatric disorders. *Epidemiologic Reviews, 19,* 144–155. http://doi.org/10.1093/oxfordjournals.epirev.a017937

Mickalak, J., Holz, A., & Teismann, T. (2011). Rumination as a predictor of relapse in mindfulness-based cognitive therapy for depression. *Psychology and Psychotherapy, 84*(2), 230–236. http://doi.org/10.1348/147608310X520166

Michalak, J., Schultze, M., Heidenreich, T., & Schramm, E. (2015). A randomized controlled trial on the efficacy of mindfulness-based cognitive therapy and a group version of cognitive behavioral analysis system of psychotherapy for chronically depressed patients. *Journal of Consulting and Clinical Psychology, 83*(5), 951–963.

Miranda, J., Azocar, F., Organista, K. C., Dwyer, E., & Areane, P. (2003). Treatment of depression among impoverished primary care patients from ethnic minority groups. *Psychiatric Services, 54*(2), 219–225. http://doi.org/10.1176/appi.ps.54.2.219

Mitani, H., Shirayama, Y., Yamada, T., Maeda, K., Ashby, C. R., & Kawahara, R. (2006). Correlation between plasma levels of glutamate, alanine and serine with severity of depression. *Progress in Neuro-Psychopharmacology and Biological Psychiatry, 30*(6), 1155–1158. http://doi.org/10.1016/j.pnpbp.2006.03.036

Montgomery, S. A., & Asberg, M. (1979). A new depression scale designed to be sensitive to change. *British Journal of Psychiatry, 134,* 382–389. http://doi.org/10.1192/bjp.134.4.382

Moore, R. G., & Garland, A. (2003). *Cognitive therapy for chronic and persistent depression.* Chichester, UK: Wiley. http://doi.org/10.1002/9780470713495

National Collaborating Centre for Mental Health. (2010). *Depression: The treatment and management of depression in adults* (Updated edition). British Psychological Society. Leicester, UK: NICE Clinical Guidelines.

Negt, P., Brakemeier, E. L., Michalak, J., Winter, L., Bleich, S., & Kahl, K. G. (2016). The treatment of chronic depression with cognitive behavioral analysis system of psychotherapy: A systematic review and meta-analysis of randomized-controlled clinical trials. *Brain and Behavior, 6*(8), e00486.

Nemeroff, C. B., Heim, C. M., Thase, M. E., Klein, D. N., Rush, A. J., Schatzberg, A. F., ... Keller, M. B. (2003). Differential responses to psychotherapy versus pharmacotherapy in patients with chronic forms of major depression and childhood trauma. *Proceedings of the National Academy of Sciences USA, 100,* 14293–14296.

Nemoto, T., Bodeker, B., & Iwamoto, M. (2011). Social support, exposure to violence, and transphobia: Correlates of depression among male-to-female transgender women with a history of sex work. *American Journal of Public Health, 101,* 1980–1988. http://doi.org/10.2105/AJPH.2010.197285

Nestler, E. J., Barrot, M., DiLeone, R. J., Eisch, A. J., Gold, S. J., & Monteggia, L. M. (2002). Neurobiology of depression. *Neuron, 34,* 13–25. http://doi.org/10.1016/S0896-6273(02)00653-0

Noble, R. E. (2005). Depression in women. *Metabolism, 54*(5 Suppl 1), 49–52. http://doi.org/10.1016/j.metabol.2005.01.014

Nuttbrock, L., Bockting, W., Rosenblum, A., Hwahng, S., Mason, M., Macri, M., ... Becker, J. (2014). Gender abuse and major depression among transgender women: A prospective study of vulnerability and resilience. *American Journal of Public Health, 104*(11), 2191–2198. http://doi.org/10.2105/AJPH.2013.301545

Nuttbrock, L., Hwahng, S., Bockting, W., Rosenblum, A., Mason, M., Macri, M., ... Becker, J. (2010). Psychiatric impact of gender-related abuse across the life course of male-to-female transgender persons. *Journal of Sex Research, 47,* 12–23. http://doi.org/10.1080/00224490903062258

Padesky, C. A. (1994). Schema change processes in cognitive therapy. *Clinical Psychology and Psychotherapy, 1*(5), 267–278. http://doi.org/10.1002/cpp.5640010502

Penberthy, J. K., Khanna, S., Lynch, M., Chhabra, D., Turk, M., Xu, Y., ... Gioia. C. (2017). Effective treatment for co-occurring alcohol use disorder and persistent. Depression: A case report. *MOJ Addiction Medicine and Therapy, 3*(3), 00035.

Persons, J. B. (1989). *Cognitive therapy in practice: A case formulation approach.* New York, NY: W. W. Norton.

Persons, J. B., & Bertagnolli, A. (1999). Inter-Rater reliability of cognitive-behavioral case formulations of depression: A replication. *Cognitive Therapy and Research, 23*(3), 271–283. http://doi.org/10.1023/A:1018791531158

Peterson, C., Semmel, A., von Baeyer, C., & Seligman, M. P. (1982). The Attributional Style Questionnaire. *Cognitive Therapy and Research, 6*(3), 287–299. http://doi.org/10.1007/BF01173577

Pettit, J. W., & Joiner, T. E. (2005). *The interpersonal solution to depression: A workbook for changing how you feel by changing how you relate.* Oakland, CA: New Harbinger.

Piccinelli, M., & Gomez Homen, F. (1997). *Gender differences in the epidemiology of affective disorders and schizophrenia.* Geneva, Switzerland: World Health Organization.

Price, J. L., & Drevets, W. C. (2012). Neural circuits underlying the pathophysiology of mood disorders. *Trends in Cognitive Science, 16*(1), 61–71. http://doi.org/10.1016/j.tics.2011.12.011

Rehm, L. P. (1977). A self-control model of depression. *Behavior Therapy, 8*(5), 787–804. http://doi.org/10.1016/S0005-7894(77)80150-0

Reilly, T. J., MacGillivray, S. A., Reid, I. C., & Cameron, I. M. (2015). Psychometric properties of the 16-item Quick Inventory of Depressive Symptomatology: A systematic review and meta-analysis. *Journal of Psychiatric Research, 60,* 132–140. http://doi.org/10.1016/j.jpsychires.2014.09.008

Renner, F., Arntz, A., Leeuw, I., & Huibers, M. (2013). Treatment for chronic depression using schema therapy. *Clinical Psychology Science and Practice, 20*(2), 166–180. http://doi.org/10.1111/cpsp.12032

Renner, F., DeRubeis, R., Arntz, A., Peeters, F., Lobbestael, J., & Huibers, M. J. (2018). Exploring mechanisms of change in schema therapy for chronic depression. *Journal of Behavioral Therapy and Experimental Psychiatry, 58,* 97–105. http://doi.org/10.1016/j.jbtep.2017.10.002

Reynolds, R. F., Dew, M. A., Pollock, B. G., Mulsant, B. H., Frank, E., Miller, M. D., … Kupfer, M. D. (2006). Maintenance treatment of major depression in old age. *New England Journal of Medicine, 354,* 1130–1138. http://doi.org/10.1056/NEJMoa052619

Reynolds, R. F., Frank, E., Perel, J. M., Imber, S. D., Cornes, C., Miller, M. D., … Kupfer, D. J. (1999). Nortriptyline and interpersonal psychotherapy as maintenance therapies for recurrent major depression: A randomized controlled trial in patients older than 59 years. *Journal of the American Medical Association, 281*(1), 39–45.

Rhebergen, D., & Graham, R. (2014). The re-labeling of dysthymic disorder to persistent depressive disorder in DSM-5: Old wine in new bottles? *Current Opinions in Psychiatry, 27,* 27–31.

Riolo, S. A., Nguyen, T., Greden, J. F., & King, C. A. (2005). Prevalence of depression by race/ethnicity: Findings from the National Health and Nutrition Examination Survey III. *American Journal of Public Health, 95*(6), 998–1000. http://doi.org/10.2105/AJPH.2004.047225

Riso, L. P., & Newman, C. F. (2003). Cognitive therapy for chronic depression. *Journal of Clinical Psychology, 59*(8), 817–831. http://doi.org/10.1002/jclp.10175

Rossello, J., Bernal, G., & Rivera-Medina, C. (2008). Individual and group CBT and IPT for Puerto Rican adolescents with depressive symptoms. *Cultural Diversity and Ethnic Minority Psychology, 14*(3), 234–245. http://doi.org/10.1037/1099-9809.14.3.234

Rossom, R. C., Shortreed, S., Coleman, K. J., Beck, A., Waitzfelder, B. E., Stewart, C., … Simon, G. E. (2016). Antidepressant adherence across diverse populations and healthcare settings. *Depression and Anxiety, 33,* 765A–774A. http://doi.org/10.1002/da.22532

Rothschild, L., & Zimmerman, M. (2002). Personality disorders and the duration of depressive episode: A retrospective study. *Journal of Personality Disorders, 16*(4), 293–303. http://doi.org/10.1521/pedi.16.4.293.24129

Rubio, J., Markowitz, J. C., & Alegria, A. (2011). Epidemiology of chronic and nonchronic major depressive disorder: Results from the national epidemiologic survey on alcohol and related conditions. *Depression and Anxiety, 28,* 622–631. http://doi.org/10.1002/da.20864

Rush, A. J., Trivedi, M. H., Ibrahim, H. M., Carmody, T. J., Arnow, B., Klein, D. N., … Keller, M. B. (2003). The 16-Item Quick Inventory of Depressive Symptomatology (QIDS), clinician rating (QIDS-C), and self-report (QIDS-SR): A psychometric evaluation in patients with chronic major depression. *Biological Psychiatry, 54*(5), 573–583.

Rush, A. J., Trivedi, M. H., Wisniewski, S. R., Nierenberg, A. A., Stewart, J. W., Warden, D., … Fava, M. (2006). Acute and longer-term outcomes in depressed outpatients requiring one or several treatment steps: A STAR*D report. *American Journal of Psychiatry, 163,* 1905–1917.

Sackeim, H. A. (2001). The definition and meaning of treatment-resistant depression. *Journal of Clinical Psychiatry, 62*(s16), 10–17.

Saltiel, P. F., & Silvershein, D. I. (2015). Major depressive disorder: Mechanism-based prescribing for personalized medicine. *Neuropsychiatric Disease and Treatment, 11,* 875–888.

Sansone, R. A., & Sansone, L. A. (2009). Early- versus late-onset dysthymia: A meaningful clinical distinction? *Psychiatry, 6*(11), 14–17.

Santiago, N. J., Klein, D. N., Vivian, D., Arnow, B. A., Blalock, J. A., Kocsis, J. H., … Keller, M. B. (2005). The therapeutic alliance and CBASP-specific skill acquisition in the treatment of chronic depression. *Cognitive Therapy and Research, 29*(6), 803–817. http://doi.org/10.1007/s10608-005-9638-5

Satyanarayana, S., Enns, M. W., Cox, B. J., & Sareen, J. (2009). Prevalence and correlates of chronic depression in the Canadian community health survey: Mental health and well-being. *Canadian Journal of Psychiatry, 54*(6), 389–398. http://doi.org/10.1177/0706743 70905400606

Schatzberg, A. F., Rush, A. J., Arnow, B. A., Banks, B. A., Blalock, J. A., Borian, F. E., … Keller, M. B. (2005). Chronic depression: Medication (nefazodone) or psychotherapy (CBASP) is effective when the other is not. *Archives of General Psychiatry, 62*(5), 513–520.

Schramm, E., Zobel, I., Dykierek, P., Kech, S., Brakemeier, E. L., Külz, A., … Berger, M. (2011). Cognitive behavioral analysis system of psychotherapy versus interpersonal psychotherapy for early-onset chronic depression: A randomized pilot study. *Journal of Affective Disorders, 129*, 109–116.

Scott, J., Teasdale, J. D., Paykel, E. S., Johnson, A. L., Abbott, R., Hayhurst, H., … Garland, A. (2000). Effects of cognitive therapy on psychological symptoms and social functioning in residual depression. *British Journal of Psychiatry, 177*(5), 440–446. http://doi.org/10.1192/bjp.177.5.440

Scottish Intercollegiate Guidelines Network. (2011). *SIGN 50: A guideline developer's handbook.* Scottish Intercollegiate Guidelines Network: Edinburgh, UK.

Segal, Z. V., Williams, J. M., & Teasdale, J. D. (2013). *Mindfulness-based cognitive therapy for depression* (2nd ed.). New York, NY: Guildford Press.

Seligman, M. E. (1973). Learned helplessness. *Annual Review of Medicine, 23*, 407–412. http://doi.org/10.1146/annurev.me.23.020172.002203

Shear, M. K., Greeno, C., Kang, J., Ludewig, D., Frank, E., Swartz, H. A., … Hanekamp, M. (2000). Diagnosis of nonpsychotic patients in community clinics. *American Journal of Psychiatry, 157*(4), 581–587. http://doi.org/10.1176/appi.ajp.157.4.581

Sheehan, D. V. (2015). *Mini International Neuropsychiatric Interview English version 7.0.0 for DSM-5.* Lyon, France: Mapi Research Trust.

Sheehan, D. V., Lecrubier, Y., Sheehan, K. H., Amorim, P., Janavs, J., Weiller, E., … Dunbar, G. C. (1998). The Mini-International Neuropsychiatric Interview (MINI): The development and validation of a structured diagnostic psychiatric interview for DSM-IV and ICD-10. *Journal of Clinical Psychiatry, 59*(Suppl 20), 22–33.

Sobell, L. C., & Sobell, M. B. (2000). Alcohol Timeline Followback (TLFB). In *Handbook of psychiatric measures* (pp. 477–479). Washington, DC: American Psychiatric Association.

Sokero, T. P., Melartin, T. K., Rytsala, H. J., Leskela, U. S., Lestela-Mielonen, P. S., & Isometsa, E. T. (2005). Prospective study of risk factors for attempted suicide among patients with DSM-IV major depressive disorder. *British Journal of Psychiatry, 186*(4), 314T–318T.

Spitzer, R. L., Endicott, J., & Robins, E. (1975). Research diagnostic criteria. *Psychopharmacology Bulletin, 11*(3), 22–25.

Spitzer, R. L., Endicott, J., & Robins, E. (1978). Research diagnostic criteria: Rationale and reliability. *Archives of General Psychiatry, 35*(6), 773–782. http://doi.org/10.1001/archpsyc.1978.01770300115013

Spitzer, R. L., Kroenke, K., Williams, J. B., & Patient Health Questionnaire Study Group. (1999). Validity and utility of a self-report version of PRIME-MD: The PHQ Primary Care Study. *Journal of the American Medical Association, 282*, 1737–1744. http://doi.org/10.1001/jama.282.18.1737

Stegenga, B. T., Kamphuis, M. H., Nazareth, I., & Geerlings, M. I. (2012). The natural course and outcome of major depressive disorder in primary care: The PREDICT-NL study. *Social Psychiatry and Psychiatric Epidemiology, 47*(1), 87–95. http://doi.org/10.1007/s00127-010-0317-9

Strik, J. J., Honig, A., Lousberg, R., & Denollet, J. (2001). Sensitivity and specificity of observer and self-report questionnaires in major and minor depression following myocardial infarction. *Psychosomatics, 42,* 423–428. http://doi.org/10.1176/appi.psy.42.5.423

Sudak, D. M. (2012). Cognitive therapy for depression. *Psychiatric Clinics of North America, 35*(1), 99–110. http://doi.org/10.1016/j.psc.2011.10.001

Swan, J. & Liebing-Wilson, M. (2018). *CBASP case formulation worksheets.* Unpublished training manuscripts.

Swan, J., Liebing-Wilson, M., MacVicar, R., & Sloan, G. (2016). Case formulation in cognitive behavioural analysis system of psychotherapy (CBASP): A case study. *British Journal of Mental Health Nursing, 5*(5), 232–241. http://doi.org/10.12968/bjmh.2016.5.5.232

Swenson, C. J., Baxter, J., Shetterly, S. M., Scarbro, S. L., & Hamman, R. F. (2000). Depressive symptoms in Hispanic and non-Hispanic White rural elderly: The San Luis Valley Health and Aging Study. *American Journal of Epidemiology, 152*(11), 1048–1055. http://doi.org/10.1093/aje/152.11.1048

Teasdale, J. D., Segal, Z. V., & Williams, J. M. (1995). How does cognitive therapy prevent relapse and why should attentional control (mindfulness) training help? *Behaviour Research and Therapy, 33,* 225–239.

Teasdale, J. D., Segal, Z. V., Williams, J. M., Ridgeway, V. A., Soulsby, J. M., & Lau, M. A. (2000). Prevention of relapse/recurrence in major depression by mindfulness-based cognitive therapy. *Journal of Consulting and Clinical Psychology, 68,* 615–623. http://doi.org/10.1037/0022-006X.68.4.615

Thaipisuttikul, P., Ittasaku, P., Waleeprakhon, P., Wisajun, P., & Jullagate, S. (2014). Psychiatric comorbidities in patients with major depressive disorder. *Neuropsychiatric Disease and Treatment, 10,* 2097–2103.

Thase, M. E., Friedman, E. S., & Howland, R. H. (2001). Management of treatment-resistant depression: Psychotherapeutic perspectives. *Journal of Clinical Psychiatry, 62*(Suppl 18), 18–24.

Thase, M. E., Greenhouse, J. B., Frank, E., Reynolds, C. F., Pilkonis, P. A., Hurley, K., … Kupfer, D. J. (1997). Treatment of major depression with psychotherapy or psychotherapy-pharmacotherapy combinations. *Archives of General Psychiatry, 54*(11), 1009–1015. http://doi.org/10.1001/archpsyc.1997.01830230043006

Tolin, D. F. (2010). Is cognitive-behavioral therapy more effective than other therapies? A meta-analytic review. *Clinical Psychology Review, 30,* 710–720. http://doi.org/10.1016/j.cpr.2010.05.003

Tolin, D. F., Gilliam, C., Wootton, B. M., Bowe, W., Bragdon, L. B., Davis, E., …Hallion, L. S. (2016). Psychometric properties of a structured diagnostic interview for DSM-5 anxiety, mood, and obsessive-compulsive and related disorders. *Assessment, 25*(1), 3–13.

Torpey, D. C., & Klein, D. N. (2008). Chronic depression: Update on classification and treatment. *Current Psychiatric Reports, 10*(6), 458–464. http://doi.org/10.1007/s11920-008-0074-6

Tsankova, N., Renthal, W., Kumar, A., & Nestler, A. J. (2007). Epigenetic regulation in psychiatric disorders. *Nature Reviews Neuroscience, 8*(5), 355–367. http://doi.org/10.1038/nrn2132

Tyrka, A. R., Wyche, M. C., Kelly, M. M., Price, L. H., & Carpenter, L. L. (2009). Childhood maltreatment and adult personality disorder symptoms: Influence of maltreatment type. *Psychiatry Research, 165*(3), 281–287. http://doi.org/10.1016/j.psychres.2007.10.017

Uher, R. (2011). Genes, environment, and individual differences in responding to treatment for depression. *Harvard Review of Psychiatry, 10,* 109–124. http://doi.org/10.3109/10673229.2011.586551

van der Velden, A. M., Kuyken, W., Wattar, U., Crane, C., Pallesen, K. J., Dahlgaard, J., … Piet, J. (2015). A systematic review of mechanisms of change in mindfulness-based cognitive therapy in the treatment of recurrent major depressive disorder. *Clinical Psychology Review, 37,* 26–39.

Vandeleur, C. L., Fassassi, S., Castelo, E., Glaus, J., Strippoli, M. F., Lasserre, A. M., ... Preisig, M. (2017). Prevalence and correlates of DSM-5 major depressive and related disorders in the community. *Psychiatry Research, 250,* 50–58. http://doi.org/10.1016/j.psychres.2017.01.060

Versiani, M., Amrein, R., Stabl, M., & International Collaborative Study Group. (1997). Moclobemide and imipramine in chronic depression (dysthymia): An international double-blind, placebo-controlled trial. *International Clinical Psychopharmacology, 12*(4), 183–194.

Viktorin, A., Lichtenstein, P., Thase, M. E., Larsson, H., Lundholm, C., Magnusson, P. K., … Landén, M. (2014). The risk of switch to mania in patients with bipolar disorder during treatment with an antidepressant alone and in combination with a mood stabilizer. *American Journal of Psychiatry, 171*(10), 1067–1073.

Vilgis, V., Chin, J., Silk, T. J., Cunnington, R., & Vance, A. (2014). Frontoparietal function in young people with dysthymic disorder (DSM-5: Persistent depressive disorder) during spatial working memory. *Journal of Affective Disorders, 160,* 34–42. http://doi.org/10.1016/j.jad.2014.01.024

Wampold, B.E., Minami, T., Baskin, T. W., Callen Tierney, S. (2002). A meta-analysis of the effects of cognitive therapy versus "other therapies" for depression. *Journal of Affective Disorders, 68,* 159–165. http://doi.org/10.1016/S0165-0327(00)00287-1

Wang, Y. P., & Gorenstein, C. (2013). Psychometric properties of the Beck Depression Inventory-II: A comprehensive review. *Revista Brasileira de Psiquiatria, 35*(4), 416–431. http://doi.org/10.1590/1516-4446-2012-1048

Waraich, P., Goldner, E. M., Somers, J. M., & Hsu, L. (2004). Prevalence and incidence studies of mood disorders: A systematic review of the literature. *Canadian Journal of Psychiatry, 49,* 124–138. http://doi.org/10.1177/070674370404900208

Warden, D., Rush, A. J., Trivedi, M. H., Fava, M., & Wisniewski, S. R. (2007). The STAR*D Project results: A comprehensive review of findings. *Current Psychiatry Reports, 9*(6), 449–459. http://doi.org/10.1007/s11920-007-0061-3

Weissman, A. N., & Beck, A. T. (1978). *Development and validation of the dysfunctional attitude scale.* Paper presented at the annual meeting of the Association for the Advanced Behavior Therapy. Chicago, IL: AABT.

Weissman, M. M., & Bothwell, S. (1976). Assessment of social adjustment by patient self-report. *Archives of General Psychiatry, 33,* 1111–1115. http://doi.org/10.1001/archpsyc.1976.01770090101010

Westra, H. A. (2004). Managing resistance in cognitive behavioural therapy: The application of motivational interviewing in mixed anxiety and depression. *Cognitive Behaviour Therapy, 33*(4), 161–175. http://doi.org/10.1080/16506070410026426

Williams, L. M., Debattista, C., Duchemin, A. M., Schatzberg, A. F., & Nemeroff, C. B. (2016). Childhood trauma predicts antidepressant response in adults with major depression: Data from the randomized international study to predict optimized treatment for depression. *Translational Psychiatry, 6*(5), e799.

Wolfe, K. L., Nakonezny, P. A., Owen, V. J., Rial, K. V., Moorehead, A. P., Kennard, B. D., … Emslie, G. J. (2017). Hopelessness as a predictor of suicide ideation in depressed male and female adolescent youth. *Suicide and Life-Threatening Behaviors, 49*(1). http://doi.org/10.1111/sltb.12428

Wong, M. I., Kling, M. A., Munson, P. J., Listwak, S., Licinio, J., Prolo, P., … Gold, P. W. (2000). Pronounced and sustained central hyper-noradrenergic function in major depression with melancholic features: Relation to hypercortisolism and corticotropin-releasing hormone. *Proceedings of the National Academy of Sciences USA, 97,* 325–330.

World Health Organization. (1992). *ICD-10 classification of mental and behavioral disorders diagnostic criteria for research.* Geneva, Switzerland: Author.

World Health Organization. (2017). *Depression and other common mental disorders*: Global Health Estimates. Geneva, Switzerland: Author.

World Health Organization. (2018). *International classification of diseases for mortality and morbidity statistics* (11th ed., stable version for implementation). Geneva, Switzerland: Author. Retrieved from https://icd.who.int/browse11/l-m/en

Young, J. E., Klosko, J. S., & Weishaar, M. E. (2003). *Schema therapy: A practitioner's guide.* New York, NY: Guilford Press.

Zanarini, M. C., Skodol, A. E., Bender, D., Dolan, R., Sanislow, C., Schaefer, E., … Gunderson, J. G. (2000). The Collaborative Longitudinal Personality Disorders Study: Reliability of axis I and II diagnoses. *Journal of Personality Disorders, 14*(4), 291–299. http://doi.org/10.1521/pedi.2000.14.4.291

Zisook, S., Lesser, I., Stewart, J. W., Wisniewski, S. R., Balasubramani, G. K., Fava, M., … Rush, A. J. (2007). Effect of age at onset on the course of major depressive disorder. *American Journal of Psychiatry, 164*(10), 1539–1546. http://doi.org/10.1176/appi.ajp.2007.06101757

Zung, W. W. (1974). Zung Self-Rating Depression Scale and Depression Status Inventory. In N. Sartorius &. T. A. Ban (Eds.), *Assessment and depression* (pp. 221–231). New York, NY: Springer Link.

7

Appendix: Tools and Resources

CBASP Significant Other History: Guide for Elicitation

Step 1
Request a list of three to five significant others who have played a major role and had a significant influence on the direction the patient's life has taken or who have shaped the individual to be who they are. The influences may be either positive or negative.

Step 2
Go through the list in the order the individuals were listed. If the list is too lengthy (i.e., greater than six or seven), ask the patient to pick the most influential five individuals.

Step 3
Begin with this question: What was it like growing up or being around this person?
Let the patient recall several memories, situations, or stories. Then, go to one of the prompts below and say:

Prompt 1.
Tell me how this person has influenced you to be the kind of person you are now.

or

Prompt 2:
How has growing up with/around this person influenced the direction your life has taken? – What is the direction?

or

Prompt 3:
What kind of a person are you as a result of living around this person? How has this person left a "stamp" on you, and what is it?

Step 4
The goal of this step is to have the patient formulate one *causal theory* conclusion for each significant other. The conclusion should represent the "stamp" or "legacy" that the patient feels the significant other has left on them that influenced the patient to be who they are now. This will take the form of a causal statement such as "because my father treated me with contempt and anger and was physically abusive, I learned that men will hurt me" or "growing up with a mother who told me she never wanted me and ignored my needs, I learned that others are not there for me."

Note: This is a Piagetian mismatching exercise, meaning that the therapist asks the preoperational patient to think and function on an abstract level here – that is, take a step back and think about the influence the significant other has had on the patient.

CBASP Case Formulation Sample Worksheet of Patient Allison D.

Allison D. is a 32-year-old woman who presented for treatment for persistent depression stating that she had always been depressed, and she reported that she thinks it is getting worse. She also has a history of alcohol abuse. She has been sober for 10 years and does not want to relapse. Allison reported that she does not remember much of her childhood. Her mother, who was also depressed, died when Allison was 10 years old, and this is when Allison thinks she realized her own depression. Allison's father was an alcoholic who became unpredictable when he was drunk. She has some memories of him being sexually inappropriate with her and exposing himself to her, but she does not remember if there was additional abuse. Her father introduced her to alcohol, giving her liquor when she was 13. She soon began to use it to "numb" her feelings of sadness, and by age 14 she was abusing alcohol regularly. At age 16, Allison moved in with her paternal grandparents when her father was sent for treatment of his addiction. She reported some improvement in both depressive symptoms and her drinking behavior, improvements which persisted until the death of her grandparents when she was 22. Allison stated that although she stopped drinking around age 17, her depression never fully improved, and when her grandparents died, she became severely depressed again but has been able to stay sober. Allison provided a significant other history with her mother, father, grandparents, and one close school friend, who moved away without telling her goodbye. Interpersonally, she appears to have difficulty getting close to people (intimacy domain), having experienced repeated loss and disappointment. She comes across to the therapist as interpersonally avoidant and distant. Allison is currently unemployed after being downsized at her job and is looking for work. She endorsed feeling depressed, lonely, and lethargic. She does not have any social support and avoids people. She does not enjoy looking for work and is not searching very hard but knows that her unemployment benefits will run out soon. She endorsed feeling severely depressed and scored 23 on the HDRS.

Presenting or Key Problems of Living
1. Depressed affect, low mood, avoidant, lethargy
2. Estranged from family and loved ones
3. Unemployed

Clinical Course Profile With Timeline for Onset, Remission, and Relapse

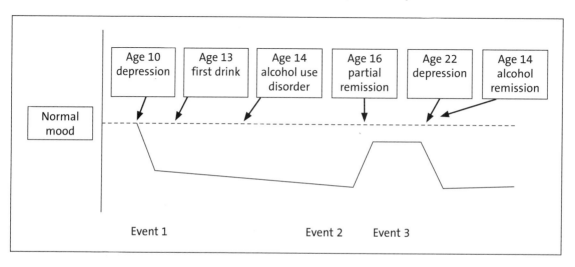

From: J. K. Penberthy: *Persistent Depressive Disorders*   © 2019 Hogrefe Publishing

Clinical course of depressive symptoms as well as symptoms of co-occurring disorders are charted on the timeline. Substance use data are captured in the boxes above to distinguish them from depressive symptoms. Start at the left with age of onset and underpin with estimations of duration for each phase of the pattern derived. You can annotate dates or other important information that best serves your purpose. You can also note these below:

Age of onset of diagnosed disorder	Trigger/timing event 1: Onset of disorder	Trigger/timing event 2: Remission of disorder	Trigger/timing Event 3: Relapse of disorder
Depression: 10 years old	Death of mother	Patient moved in with grandparents	Death of grandparents
Alcohol use disorder: 14 years old	Father introduces alcohol	Grandparents placed father in treatment for alcoholism	Patient leaves grandparents' home

Significant Other History (SOH)

Significant other	Causal theory conclusion (stamp)
Mother	"Positive relationships don't last."
Father	"Men are dangerous and confusing, I can't trust them."
Grandparents	"Good people can only do so much, and they don't last."
Friend	"Getting close to people only leads to disappointment and pain."

Transference Hypothesis

Domain	Transference hypothesis
Intimacy	"If I get close to Dr. Penberthy, she will leave me or hurt me."
Making mistakes	
Expressing negative affect	
Expressing needs	

Ideally, try to construct at least one transference hypothesis as it may apply to the relationship between the therapist and the patient.

From: J. K. Penberthy: *Persistent Depressive Disorders*   © 2019 Hogrefe Publishing

Impact Message Inventory

The therapist completes the Impact Message Inventory (IMI) based on interpersonal reactions to the patient and graphs the scores on the circumplex to help inform the relationship with the patient. DOM = dominant; FRI-DOM = friendly–dominant; FRI = friendly; FRI-SUB = friendly–submissive; SUB = submissive; HOS-SUB = hostile–submissive; HOS = hostile; HOS-DOM = hostile–dominant.

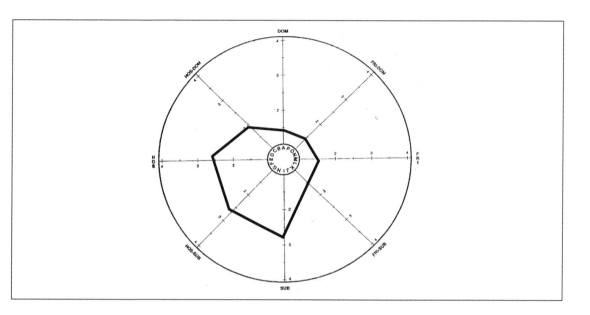

Patient's actual stimulus values (peaks on IMI)	Description of actual problematic behavior in the interpersonal environment	Potential interpersonal response and consequence with the therapist	Potential interpersonal response and consequence outside therapy
Hostile	• Avoiding people or being short with people, not looking them in the eye	→ Therapist feels distant from Allison and is pulled to be hostile in return	→ People respond in a hostile way and stay away from Allison or ignore her
Hostile-submissive	• Expressing strong negative feelings and hopelessness to others repeatedly	→ Therapist wants to help, but finds Allison hard to approach, so wants to take charge of the session	→ People cannot get close to Allison and tell her what they think she should do, or they get fed up and withdraw from her
Submissive	• Going along with what other people suggest. Allison does not voice her needs or preferences	→ Therapist takes control when Allison can't make up her mind about what to do or talk about	→ Others don't see what Allison wants, and assume she is happy to do go along

From: J. K. Penberthy: *Persistent Depressive Disorders*   © 2019 Hogrefe Publishing

CBASP Case Formulation Worksheet

Patient: _____ Therapist: _____ Date: _____

Presenting or Key Problems of Living
(Brief description in order of priority or importance or impact.)

1. _____

2. _____

3. _____

4. _____

Clinical Course Profile

From information developed from the timeline, you should sketch out the clinical course profile that best captures the course of the patient's experience of depression. Start at the left with age of onset and record duration for each phase of the pattern below the line. You can annotate dates or other important information for your purposes. You can also note onset and events (remission, relapse, etc.) in the following table:

Age of onset	Trigger/timing event 1	Trigger/timing event 2	Trigger/timing event 3:

From: J. K. Penberthy: *Persistent Depressive Disorders*   © 2019 Hogrefe Publishing

Significant Other History

Significant other	Causal theory conclusion (stamp)

Transference Hypothesis

Domain	Transference hypothesis
Intimacy	
Making mistakes	
Expressing negative affect	
Expressing needs	

    Ideally, try to construct at least one transference hypothesis (TH) as it may apply to the relationship between the therapist and the patient. Clinical experience suggests this is often difficult. Therefore, it is legitimate to have more than one TH but endeavor to target the primary one.

From: J. K. Penberthy: *Persistent Depressive Disorders*   © 2019 Hogrefe Publishing

Impact Message Inventory

The therapist completes the Impact Message Inventory (IMI) based on interpersonal reactions to the patient and graphs the scores on the circumplex to help inform the relationship with the patient. DOM = dominant; FRI-DOM = friendly–dominant; FRI = friendly; FRI-SUB = friendly–submissive; SUB = submissive; HOS-SUB = hostile–submissive; HOS = hostile; HOS-DOM = hostile–dominant.

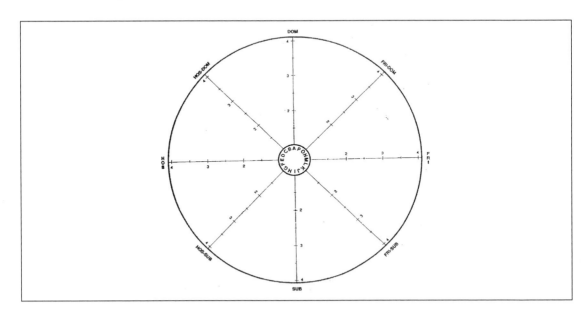

Patient's actual stimulus values (peaks on IMI)	Description of actual problematic behavior in the interpersonal environment	Potential interpersonal response and consequence with the therapist	Potential interpersonal response and consequence outside therapy

Treatment Plan

- Assessment (including timeline, significant other history, transference hypothesis, and impact message inventory)
- Introduction to situational analysis
- Situational analysis of distressing interpersonal events – one slice of time each session
- Optional – skills training (what is the one thing to add to your repertoire?)

Summary

This is written to the patient and is a summary of the patient's background, assessment outcomes, and treatment plan, as well as possible difficulties, related to their stimulus value and current behavioral repertoire.

From: J. K. Penberthy: *Persistent Depressive Disorders* © 2019 Hogrefe Publishing

CBASP Situational Analysis Format for the Coping Survey Questionnaire

Situation → Interpretations → Behaviors → Actual Outcome (AO) → Desired Outcome (DO) → AO = DO? → Why?/Why Not?

1. Describe the situation in behavioral terms (like you would a movie clip), with a beginning, middle, and end point.
   a. What happened first…
   b. In the middle…
   c. At the end…

2. Describe how you interpreted the situation, what it meant to you, what you made of it. Follow along the timeline of the situation when you give your interpretations.

   _____

   _____

3. Describe how you behaved in the situation … what you did, how you did it, what you said, how you said it, etc.

   _____

   _____

4. Describe how the event actually came out for you. This is the *actual outcome* (AO) and should be described behaviorally.

   _____

   _____

5. Describe how you wanted the event to come out for you? This is your *desired outcome* (DO) and should be a realistic and attainable (preferably interpersonal behavioral) goal.

   _____

   _____

6. Did your AO = DO? In other words, did you get what you wanted?

   YES / NO / MAYBE / NOT SURE

7. Why or why not did your AO = DO?

   _____

   _____

From: J. K. Penberthy: *Persistent Depressive Disorders*   © 2019 Hogrefe Publishing

Elicitation Phase Prompts for Situational Analysis in CBASP

Step 1
Tell me what happened in the situation. Give a beginning, middle, and end.

Step 2
Tell me what the situation meant to you or how you read it. Think back over the event, and describe what it meant to you from the beginning to the end. Give me one sentence for each interpretation.

Step 3
Think about what you did in the situation, and how you behaved or acted. Did you speak? What was your voice like? Did you make eye contact?

Step 4
Tell me how the situation came out for you. What was the *actual outcome* (AO)? Give me one sentence that describes the outcome and that an observer could see.

Step 5
Think about the outcome. How would you have liked the situation to come out for you? This is the goal or *desired outcome* (DO). Tell me in one sentence how you wanted it to come out for you. Remember, this needs to be something that you can do. The DO needs to be realistic and attainable.

Step 6
Now think about the AO and the DO.
Did you get what you wanted here?
Did the AO = the DO? YES or NO

Step 7
Why did you or didn't you obtain the desired outcome?

Reprinted with permission from unpublished material by James P. McCullough, Jr., 2018.
This page may be reproduced by the purchaser for personal/clinical use.
From: J. K. Penberthy: *Persistent Depressive Disorders*   © 2019 Hogrefe Publishing

Remediation Phase Prompts for Situational Analysis in CBASP

If you have determined that the desired outcome (DO) is not realistic (the patient cannot produce it) or not attainable (the environment cannot produce it), then the DO will need to be revised.

This can be done by asking the patient if they think that the DO is realistically achievable and working with them in a motivational interviewing, collaborative style, to help them ascertain that it may not be an appropriate DO if it is deemed something that they cannot produce or that the environment cannot produce. The therapist can let the patient come to this determination – the patient may struggle, but it will mean more if they determine that the goal they have is not feasible, and they work to modify it with you.

If it is established that the DO is not realistic or attainable, work with the patient to establish one that is. This can be done by asking, "What do you think is a realistic goal in this situation, but not the AO?" or "What might be a first step toward what you want?"

When a realistic, attainable goal is set, then the therapist can proceed to remediation. The therapist may wish to briefly review the situation again, especially if the elicitation phase has been long and complicated. Use the patient's words and terminology, and check with the patient that you have it right. When this is completed, proceed with …

Therapist: Now, let's go back into the situation and see what you might have changed to get what you wanted. The first thing we'll look at is the way you interpreted the event.

Step 1
The therapist says something similar to the below:

In your **first interpretation**, you said………. Is this interpretation grounded in the event? That is, is it based on the present event, or is it based on the past or future? (it is a *relevant interpretation*);
Do you feel that the interpretation is an accurate description of the interaction? (I mean, do you think the interpretation accurately describes what is happening between you and the other person, or something that is happening in you: feelings, thoughts, etc.);
Finally, what does this interpretation contribute toward you getting what you want? How does it help you achieve your desired outcome? (it may or may not; just so it is *relevant* and *accurate*).

In your **second interpretation**…… (go through each interpretation, which may follow the timeline of the situation).
The therapist and patient go through each interpretation, revising and eliminating portions of them until there are statements that are relevant, accurate, grounded, and helpful toward facilitating achievement of a realistic and attainable goal. If necessary the therapist may need to add interpretations and may say something like:
You need an Action Interpretation – a thought you could say to yourself that would prompt you to take action, to say what you want or don't want, etc., what could that be?

Step 2
The therapist says something similar to the below:

If you had thought of an *action interpretation*, how would your behavior have changed?
Had you behaved this way, would you have gotten what you wanted – that is, your *desired outcome*? (focus on solidifying learning)

Step 3

The therapist says something similar to the below:

What have you learned here? (therapist focuses on solidifying learning)

Step 4

The therapist says something similar to the below:

Can you think of any other similar situation where what you have learned here can be applied? Tell me about it. (therapist focuses on generalization of learning)

 © 2019 Hogrefe Publishing

Internet Resources

Additional information and resources can be accessed through the sources and websites below. Many of these organizations can provide additional information about persistent depressive disorder (PDD) and training in their psychotherapeutic approach to treating PDD. Some require membership to access materials, but all of the websites are rich resources for information.

National Institute of Mental Health Website on Depression

https://www.nimh.nih.gov/health/publications/depression-what-you-need-to-know/index.shtml

This is an excellent website with the latest information on research in depression, including PDD. This site provides user-friendly handouts for patients regarding diagnosis of depression and other resources for help. This is a critical resource for clinicians working with depressed patients. There are informational booklets and other free materials available to download and provide to patients.

American Psychological Association

http://www.apa.org/topics/depression/

This section of the APA website focuses on depression and provides guidance for clinicians as well as information that can be downloaded and shared with patients. This is an excellent resource for user-friendly information about how to get help for depression.

Interpersonal Psychotherapy Institute

https://iptinstitute.com/about-ipt/

This organization and website provide information and training on IPT for depression and other disorders. The site includes links to materials and information helpful in learning about and conducting IPT.

Beck Institute for Cognitive Behavior Therapy

https://beckinstitute.org/get-training/

This is the training institute website for cognitive behavior therapy (CBT) and provides information about CBT for depression.

Academy of Cognitive Therapy

http://www.academyofct.org/page/TrainingPrograms

This website and training academy provides information and materials about how to become trained in CBT. Additional materials are available for members, and this site provides information about how to obtain formal training and certification.

Cognitive Behavioral Analysis System of Psychotherapy

http://www.cbasp.org/

This is James McCullough's website on CBASP and provides information about research and ongoing training opportunities, as well as on how to become certified.

CBASP Network

http://www.cbasp-network.org/

This is a German website (in German) that provides information about CBASP, current studies, and training, as well as information on conferences and happenings across Europe.

International CBASP Society

http://www.cbaspsociety.org/

This is an international organization with a website that provides information about CBASP research, providers, and ongoing training and certification opportunities. It has resources and materials available for members.

Your Guide to Mindfulness-Based Cognitive Therapy

http://mbct.com/

This website is focused on MBCT and provides additional information about research and training opportunities as well as resources for MBCT.

© 2019 Hogrefe Publishing

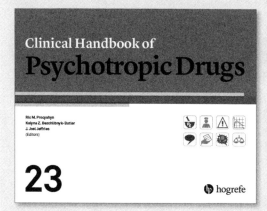

Ric M. Procyshyn / Kalyna Z. Bezchlibnyk-Butler /
J. Joel Jeffries (Editors)

Clinical Handbook of Psychotropic Drugs

23rd edition 2019, iv + 454 pp.
+ 63 pp. of printable PDF patient information sheets
US $99.80 / € 79.95
ISBN 978-0-88937-561-1
Also available as online version

The *Clinical Handbook of Psychotropic Drugs* has become a standard reference and working tool for psychiatrists, psychologists, physicians, pharmacists, nurses, and other mental health professionals.

- Packed with unique, easy-to-read comparison charts and tables (dosages, side effects, pharmacokinetics, interactions...) for a quick overview of treatment options

- Succinct, bulleted information on all classes of medication: on- and off-label indications, side effects, interactions, pharmacodynamics, precautions in the young, the elderly, and pregnancy, nursing implications, and much more – all you need to know for each class of drug

- Potential interactions and side effects summarized in comparison charts

- With instantly recognizable icons and in full color throughout, allowing you to find at a glance all the information you seek

- Clearly written patient information sheets available for download as printable PDF files

This book is a must for everyone who needs an up-to-date, easy-to-use, comprehensive summary of all the most relevant information about psychotropic drugs.

New in this edition:
- Antidepressants chapter includes a new section on the NMDA receptor antagonist esketamine (Spravato), also updates to antidepressant use in pregnancy and SPARI drug interactions

- Antipsychotics updates include a new section on 5-HT2A inverse agonist antipsychotic (pimavanserin, Nuplazid) and comprehensive revision of augmentation strategies

- Pharmacogenomics chapter fully revised with expanded dose adjustment recommendations and guidelines

- Chart of agents under investigation for treatment of substance use disorders fully revised, new agents include lofexidine (Lucemyra), Kadian, nortriptyline, e-cigarettes

- Unapproved treatments chapter with significant updates, including new sections on adrenergic agents in PTSD (doxazosin), antiflammatory agents in depression (pioglitazone, rosiglitazone, statins), and hormones in schizophrenia (raloxifene)

- Expanded treatment options for extrapyramidal side effects include deutetrabenazine and valbenazine (vesicular monoamine transporter 2 (VMAT2) inhibitors)

- New formulations and trade names include: Adzenys ER (amphetamine), Aristada (aripiprazole), Austedo (deutetrabenazine), Cotempla XR-ODT (methylphenidate), Fanatrex FusePaq (gabapentin), Foquest (methylphenidate), Ingrezza (valbenazine), Jornay PM (methylphenidate), Mydayis (mixed amphetamine salts), Nuplazid (pimavanserin), Spravato (esketamine), Sublocade (buprenorphine), Zelapar (selegiline)

www.hogrefe.com

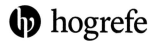

Advances in Psychotherapy
Evidence-Based Practice

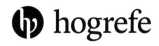

New Titles

Developed and edited with the support of the
Society of Clinical Psychology (APA Division 12)

Editors
Danny Wedding, PhD, MPH, USA
Larry E. Beutler, PhD, USA
Kenneth E. Freedland, PhD, USA
Linda Carter Sobell, PhD, ABPP, USA
David. A. Wolfe, PhD, Canada

About the series
The *Advances in Psychotherapy* series provides therapists and students with practical, evidence-based guidance on the diagnosis and treatment of the most common disorders seen in clinical practice – and does so in a uniquely reader-friendly manner. Each book is both a compact "how-to" reference on a particular disorder, for use by professional clinicians in their daily work, and an ideal educational resource for students and for practice-oriented continuing education. The books all have a similar structure, and each title is a compact and easy-to-follow guide covering all aspects of practice that are relevant in real life. Tables, boxed clinical "pearls," and marginal notes assist orientation, while checklists for copying and summary boxes provide tools for use in daily practice.

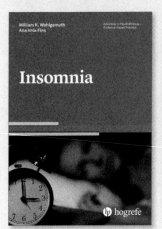

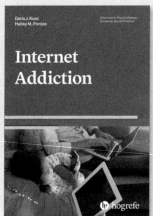

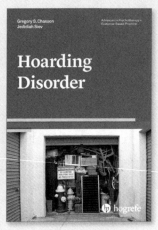

Volume 42
2019, viii + 94 pp.
ISBN 978-0-88937-415-7

Volume 41
2019, iv + 86 pp.
ISBN 978-0-88937-501-7

Volume 40
2019, viii + 76 pp.
ISBN 978-0-88937-407-2

For a list of all current volumes, see next page.

www.hogrefe.com

hogrefe

Advances in Psychotherapy

Prices: US $29.80/€ 24.95 per volume. Standing order price US $24.80/€ 19.95 per volume
(minimum 4 successive volumes) + postage & handling. Special rates for APA Division 12 and Division 42 members

www.hogrefe.com

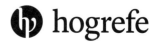 hogrefe

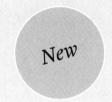
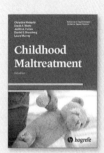
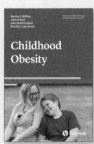
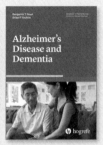
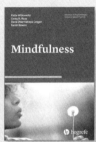
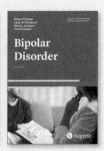
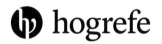

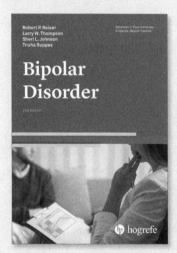
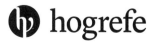

An essential reference for assessing and treating people with schizophrenia spectrum disorders

"Without question, the clearest explanation of the nature of the schizophrenia spectrum and, more importantly, what to do about it."

Joel A. Dvoskin, PhD, ABPP (Forensic), University of Arizona College of Medicine, Tucson, AZ

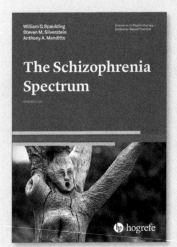

William D. Spaulding / Steven M. Silverstein / Anthony A. Menditto

The Schizophrenia Spectrum

(Series: Advances in Psychotherapy –
Evidence-Based Practice – Volume 5)
2nd edition 2017, viii + 94 pp.
US $29.80 / € 24.95
ISBN 978-0-88937-504-8
Also available as eBook

The new edition of this highly acclaimed volume provides a fully updated and comprehensive account of the psychopathology, clinical assessment, and treatment of schizophrenia spectrum disorders. It emphasizes functional assessment and modern psychological treatment and rehabilitation methods, which continue to be under-used despite overwhelming evidence that they improve outcomes. The compact and easy-to-read text provides both experienced practitioners and students with an evidence-based guide incorporating the major developments of the last decade: the new diagnostic criteria of the DSM-5, introducing the schizophrenia spectrum and neurodevelopmental disorders, the further evolution of recovery as central to treatment and rehabilitation, advances in understanding the psychopathology of schizophrenia, and the proliferation of psychological and psychosocial modalities for treatment and rehabilitation.

www.hogrefe.com

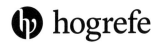